HARM LESS

a nudge to reconnect - with yourself & the planet

ARTI MISHRA

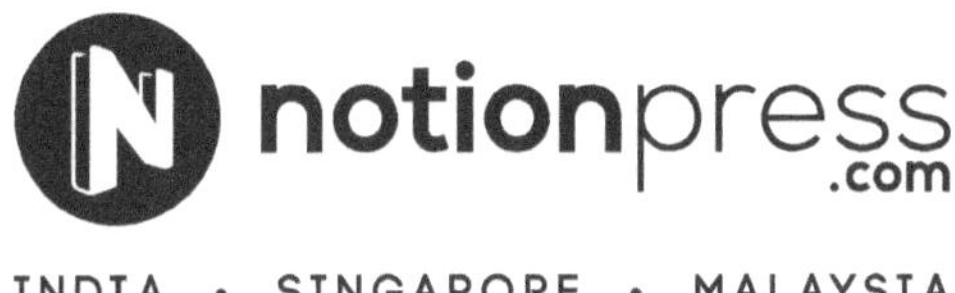

INDIA · SINGAPORE · MALAYSIA

ISBN
Paperback 979-8-89632-811-7
Hardcase 979-8-89673-812-1

Dedication

"To my father,

A soldier, a sharpshooter, and a pure soul.

From you I learned courage, fearlessness, and determination.

You were always in the fields, protecting our country, while we grew up away from you. You taught me the beauty of simplicity—how to cherish the soil, do farming, rear cows, and natural ways of living. Your love for agriculture, animals, nature and belief in living close to the earth continue to inspire me every day. Your words stayed with me: stay close to the soil, love your body, and honour the planet.

Your courage, fearless spirit, and connection to nature are a part of me now. ***HARM less*** is my humble effort to share your values with the world and inspire others to love their bodies and our planet.

This book is my tribute to you, your lessons, and the life you lived so beautifully.

With endless gratitude, love, and admiration."

Table of Contents

Foreword

It is with great pleasure and admiration that I introduce you to "***HARM less***," a profound and timely work by my dear friend Arti. Over the years, I have had the privilege of witnessing Arti's journey, one marked by a deep commitment to understanding the intricate connections between our bodies, our environment, and the choices we make every day.

From the moment I met Arti, it was clear that she possessed a unique perspective on life. Her passion for natural living and sustainability was not just a passing interest but a way of life that permeated every aspect of her being. Whether it was through her meticulous selection of natural products, her dedication to sustainable practices, or her ability to find beauty in the simplest moments of nature, Arti embodied the principles of "***HARM less***" long before this book took shape.

"***HARM less***" is the culmination of Arti's years of exploration, research, and personal experience. It is a heartfelt invitation to slow down, reconnect with the natural world, and rediscover the wisdom our ancestors once held dear. Through eloquent storytelling and practical advice, Arti guides us on a journey that is both enlightening and transformative.

In these pages, you will find a wealth of insights that bridge the gap between the past and the present. Arti takes us back to a time when life was in harmony with nature and then leads us through the complexities of the modern world, where synthetic products and convenience have often overshadowed sustainability and well-being. With a keen eye for detail and a compassionate heart, Arti unravels the hidden impacts of our daily choices, urging us to awaken to the realities of our chemical-laden world.

What makes "***HARM less***" truly special is its holistic approach. Arti seamlessly blends scientific concepts like entropy with practical steps for reducing our environmental footprint. Each chapter is a gentle reminder that our actions, no matter how small, have the power to create ripples of positive change. From natural skincare routines to sustainable dietary practices, Arti offers a wealth of knowledge that empowers us to make mindful choices that benefit both our health and the planet.

As you read "***HARM less***," you will feel Arti's passion and dedication in every word. Her journey is a testament to the power of living with intention and respect for the world around us. This book is a call to action, a reminder that we can restore balance and harmony in our lives and in our environment.

I am incredibly proud of Arti and the work she has created. "***HARM less***" is a gift to all who seek a deeper connection with nature and a more sustainable way of living. It is a beacon of hope in a world that often feels disconnected and chaotic. As you embark on this journey, may you find inspiration, peace, and a renewed sense of purpose.

Welcome to the world of ***HARM less.***

—Sheril Christopher

BE | Environment Engineer & PG | Industrial Safety

From Visvesvaraya Technological University

Introduction

Pause for a moment, take a deep breath in, exhale slowly, and think about this: you wake up one morning, and the sunlight softly filters through the windows. As you step outside, the cool earth beneath your feet grounds you, and the fresh, crisp air fills your lungs. The world is alive with the gentle sound of leaves rustling, and the songs of birds fill the air, greeting you as a new day begins. In this calm moment, you notice everything around you: the bright colors of nature, the soft breeze flowing through the branches, and the light scent of blooming flowers.

Standing there, you feel your heartbeat, steady and calm, almost in rhythm with the life around you. Each breath you take feels connected to everything, reminding you that you belong to something bigger. It's easy to get caught up in the rush of everyday life and forget these simple moments. Yet, in this peaceful setting, it becomes clear: your body isn't just here to get you through the day. It deserves care and attention, like a temple where your spirit finds peace and strength when treated with the same respect as the world around you.

As you take in that peaceful moment, it's worth reflecting on the words of Jim Rohn, who once said, *"Treat your body like a temple, not a woodshed."* Closer to home, the renowned yoga teacher B.K.S. Iyengar also shared a similar thought: *"The body is your temple. Keep it pure and clean for the soul to reside in."* These words offer a powerful metaphor, inviting us to think about how we care for and honor the body, much like the way we care for a sacred space.

When we view the body as a temple, the idea goes beyond simply looking after our health—it shifts how we see the world around us. This mindset naturally extends to how we treat the environment, which we can think of as the surroundings of this temple. If we hold our bodies in reverence, it's only natural that we begin to see the natural world with the same respect and care.

Nurturing our bodies and our surroundings creates a sense of peace and balance. Just as a temple offers a place of refuge and reflection, nature provides a similar sanctuary. Spending time in natural settings, practicing mindfulness, or simply being still in a quiet moment deepens our connection to ourselves and to the earth. This connection encourages us to protect and cherish the natural world, recognizing that our environment is an essential part of our existence.

The idea of treating our bodies and surroundings as sacred isn't new. My father always emphasized that you must not apply synthetic products to your body, and I've learned how to make the best use of kitchen ingredients for our body care from my mother. As I got into it, I discovered that many cultures hold this belief deeply, influencing how people live each day. In many Indigenous cultures, for instance, there is a strong sense of interconnectedness between the body and the natural world. The body is seen as a part of a larger ecosystem, where every element is closely tied together. This worldview inspires deep respect for nature, promoting rooted way of living that seeks balance with the environment. Indigenous knowledge systems often blend spiritual practices with environmental stewardship, creating a reciprocal relationship with nature. When something is taken from the earth, it is balanced by giving back, ensuring that natural resources are respected and preserved for future generations. This balance, rooted in the idea of sacredness, is a key principle that has guided these cultures for centuries.

In traditional Japanese culture, we find a similar belief through the concept of Shinto, which emphasizes purity and cleanliness—both physically and spiritually. Natural spaces like mountains, rivers, and forests are viewed as sacred, and the practice of personal cleanliness is seen as an extension of this reverence for the environment. By keeping their bodies clean, people are reminded to treat their surroundings with the same level of care and respect. It's an approach that creates a deep sense of peace and balance, where the connection between the body and the world outside it is always in focus.

In Indian culture, the idea of the body as a temple has become even more widespread through practices like yoga and mindfulness. These approaches encourage people to live consciously, paying attention to the choices they make every day. This way of living helps create a deeper connection to nature, reminding us to love and respect the earth as we nurture our bodies.

These different cultures all point to the same truth: how we treat our bodies is linked to how we treat the world around us. This is where the idea of Rooted Living comes in. Rooted Living encourages a return to a balanced way of life, making choices that honor both personal well-being and the planet. It's about embracing practices that are ***HARM less***—choices that reduce harm to our bodies while preserving the planet for generations to come. By living in alignment with this philosophy, we create a world where nature and humanity thrive together.

As I reflect on history, I'm inspired by the many cultures worldwide that embraced what I like to call "rooted living." These cultures recognized that by tapping into the resources available in their local ecosystems, they could achieve physical and mental balance.

In many Indigenous cultures, for instance, the use of native plants for medicine has been an integral part of life. These communities have a deep respect for their natural surroundings, understanding that maintaining harmony with the environment ensures both survival and well-being. Take Indigenous Australians as an example: they've long used plants like eucalyptus and tea tree oil for their healing properties. These oils are prized for their ability to cleanse and heal wounds, and Mint has been relied upon to help treat respiratory issues. These practices are living examples of how a community can stay rooted to its environment and manage its resources planet-friendly, passing this wisdom down through generations.

Similarly, the Mediterranean region has long embraced a diet rich in local herbs like rosemary, thyme, and basil, which are flavorful and known for their health benefits. The Mediterranean diet has become famous for its ability to reduce the risk of chronic diseases. But beyond the food on the plate, this way of life is rooted in a respect for the land. It relies on agricultural methods that preserve local ecosystems, showing how cultural practices are planet-friendly, promoting health for both people and the planet.

Similarly, in India, the concept of rooted living comes to life through the traditional system of Ayurveda, which translates to "the science of life." Ayurveda teaches that the key to health and well-being lies in using the natural elements around us to bring balance to both body and mind. This practice has been passed down through generations, integrating herbs, spices, and oils into daily routines as a way to maintain that balance.

Ayurveda's use of oils is another reflection of this philosophy. Practices such as abhyanga, a self-massage using these oils, are designed to nourish the skin, soothe the mind, and restore balance. These oils are often infused with herbs like neem, garlic cloves or brahmi to boost their healing properties, creating a practice that truly connects the body with nature's gifts. It's a daily ritual that serves as a reminder of the deep relationship between self-care and the environment.

India's long-standing embrace of Ayurveda shows us how cultures can look to their local ecosystems for everything needed to endure well-being. Through this integration of natural elements into everyday life, Ayurveda offers a path toward harmony—both within the body and with the world around us.

These glimpses back into history offer us a quick snapshot of how harmonious and rooted living once was. Life was closely intertwined with nature, and people relied on their immediate surroundings to care for their bodies and well-being. But let's bring this closer to home—think about your own grandparents or great-grandparents. I often think back to my childhood, spending time growing up with my parents and grandparents in our village. They had no reliance on store-bought, artificial products. Everything we used was homemade, simple, and natural. I still remember my mother washing her hair with soapnut and cleaning the floors with nothing more than water and a dash of salt or homemade liquid from lemon or orange peels. For cooking, she would use fresh produce from her kitchen garden and oils freshly done from mustard seeds in front of her eyes. I learned to pluck fresh vegetables, leafy greens, dug potatoes, ginger from soil from her. Life was different, slower in a way that felt more connected to the earth. And often without the need for products from a store.

But I saw things change faster as I grew into a school going kid and with my parents too eventually. Artificial products started creeping into our homes, and by the time I was in high school, the world had completely shifted. And now, it feels like everything is available in a bottle or box, each promising convenience but pulling us further away from those simple, natural ways of living.

Despite the beauty and richness of this concept of rooted living and viewing our bodies as temples, there's no denying the heavy disconnect in modern life. Somewhere along the way, we drifted away from these principles.

When we wonder why this is, we see that the shift has been driven by a deep-rooted change in society—one that prioritizes convenience and instant gratification over planet-friendly and long-term well-being.

Modern life is shaped by a desire for ease and efficiency, which has transformed the way we consume products. The emphasis on quick solutions and immediate results has created a culture where we reach for what's fast and convenient, often without thinking about the long-term impact. This mindset is everywhere, from the products we use on our bodies to the items we bring into our homes. The demand for convenience has led to an overwhelming dependance on artificial, mass-produced products that promise to make life easier. What we overlook or completely ignore is that it comes at the expense of our own health and our environment.

For example, take a moment to think about the products we use daily—cleaners, body washes, lotions, and more. We often choose these items for their instant benefits, without considering the complex chemicals inside them. These products offer immediate results, but what we don't see are the hidden costs. The reliance on artificial ingredients has detached us from the natural alternatives our grandparents once used, breaking the bond we once had with nature and its healing properties.

The pull of convenience in modern life is strong, and companies know how to tap into it. Through advertising, they create a picture of success and happiness that seems directly tied to consumption. From single-use plastics to fast fashion, we're bombarded with messages that make us feel like we constantly need something new. These ads make disposable goods appear glamorous, steering us away from valuing items that last.

But beneath this shiny surface lies a darker reality—the waste piles up, natural resources are drained, and the environment pays the price. This culture of constant consumption has shifted focus entirely from the deep value of nature and the importance of loving and preserving it.

Urbanization has played a big role in this change as well. As cities grow, they swallow up the natural landscapes that once surrounded us. Concrete replaces green, and access to natural spaces becomes harder to find. With fewer chances to connect with nature, many of us begin to feel distant from it. This physical separation from the natural world also creates a mental distance. We become less aware of the benefits that come from living in harmony with the environment, and more accustomed to the fast-paced, efficiency-driven lifestyle of urban living.

Then there's technology, which has further accelerated this detachment from rooted living. With the rise of mass production, synthetic goods are everywhere, and they're often marketed as better options. These products promise durability, ease of use, and affordability—qualities that seem perfect for modern life. But in doing so, they push aside the traditional, natural alternatives that our grandparents relied on. Clothing, personal care items, and household products are now made from synthetic materials, overshadowing the natural fibers and ingredients that once formed the foundation of daily life.

Technology has also changed how we interact with these products. With just a few clicks, we can have anything delivered to our door, often without thinking about where it comes from or the impact it has. E-commerce and digital marketing make it so easy to acquire more, all while the environment bears the cost. This endless cycle of consumption pushes aside the principles of quality, longevity, and sustainability, leaving us more disconnected from the natural world than ever before.

The growing disconnection between us and the natural world has created a profound divide—one that affects how we live, how we view ourselves and our place in the world. It's as though we've forgotten an essential truth: our bodies are temples, sacred and deserving of care, just as the earth itself is sacred and in need of respect. To heal this fracture, we must shift our perspective, embracing the philosophy that how we treat ourselves and how we treat the planet are deeply intertwined.

The philosophy of "Body as Temple" and rooted living teaches us that every choice we make impacts our personal well-being and the health of the environment around us. It invites us to live harmoniously with the rhythms of nature, recognizing that when we harm ourselves—through the chemicals we use, the foods we consume, or the waste we generate—we also harm the planet. Conversely, when we care for ourselves with intention, we extend that same care to the earth. This alignment creates a life that is truly ***HARM less***—for both our bodies and the world we inhabit.

In the context of this alignment, rooted living is about making thoughtful, deliberate choices that nourish and sustain. It's a call to slow down, to reconsider the products we use, the foods we eat, and the habits we've grown accustomed to, through the lens of care and respect. This approach challenges us to step away from convenience-driven habits and reconnect with a lifestyle that honors simplicity, intentionality, and the interconnectedness of all things.

The pages ahead guide you on this journey, offering insights but also practical steps to help you live in a way that aligns with these principles. The first part of this book reveals how we arrived at a place of dependency on artificial products, exploring how industrialization and marketing gradually shaped our choices, often at the expense of our health and the environment. This understanding is crucial—it helps you see the hidden forces at play and empowers you to reclaim control over your decisions.

As you move through these pages, you'll find practical steps and natural alternatives that can help you live more intentionally, in a way that nourishes both your body and the environment. The final part broadens the horizon, inviting you to see how your individual choices can spark a positive impact, influencing industries, policies, and even the world around you. This is where the power of rooted living extends beyond your home and into a collective movement for environmental preservation.

We are all set to begin this journey together, and I would like to share a few inspiring words from American philosopher William James at this juncture, as they speak to the heart of what we are going to explore. He once said, "Act as if what you do makes a difference. It does." These words carry a simple yet profound truth—our actions, no matter how small they seem, can have a lasting impact. And as we move forward, I want you to keep this in mind: the changes you make will touch your life and the world in ways you may not even realize.

Change, I understand, can be daunting, that hesitancy before taking the first step is natural. It's worth the effort, especially when the convenience of modern life pulls us in the opposite direction. But I can assure you, the rewards of embracing rooted living are immeasurable. Together, we'll make a difference, and I'll be right here with you as you begin to see the impact this change can have on your life and the world around you.

Section 1

The Silent Takeover: Our Chemical Reality

Chapter 1

The Chemical Invasion – How We Got Here

To grasp how we arrived at this point, let's first journey back to where it all started: the pre-industrial ages. Before the world became dominated by industry and machines, people lived in harmony with their surroundings. Life was slower, and the pace of each day was dictated by the land, the weather, and the seasons. Communities were small, often built around families or tribes, and survival meant understanding the wisdom of working with nature's rhythms—finding balance in its gifts and limits, and ensuring that every resource was used with purpose and respect. There were no factories churning out products; just humans, nature, and the knowledge passed down through generations about how to use the earth's resources wisely.

People relied on the land for their most basic needs: food, clothing, and shelter. They hunted, fished, and foraged, moving as needed when resources became scarce. This kind of life, deeply connected to the environment, required a sharp understanding of local plants, animals, and ecosystems. Tools were made from materials found in nature, such as stone, bone, and wood, and every part of an animal or plant was used with purpose and care.

As time passed, humans learned to farm, and this changed everything. Instead of moving from place to place, they began to settle. Farming meant planting crops and raising animals for food, leading to the growth of permanent villages and, eventually towns. People began to live in closer-knit communities, but even then, life remained deeply connected to nature. Agriculture shaped the rhythms of daily life, but it also relied on the earth's cycles, reinforcing a respectful relationship with the land that sustained them.

As agriculture advanced, life changed in ways that would have seemed remarkable to earlier generations. With the ability to produce surplus food, communities expanded. Populations grew, towns formed, and human societies began to take on new shapes and complexities. People who were once solely focused on survival and food gathering found the freedom to explore other activities, which led to the rise of specialized crafts and trades.

At this time, small-scale industries thrived. These were often family-run operations where goods like handlooms, pottery, furniture, leather items, metalwork, carpets, and household tools were crafted by hand or with simple machines powered by people or animals. In addition to these, materials like stone and bricks were also shaped with care and skill, contributing to the construction of homes and community spaces. Everything from wool to wood was sourced directly from the environment. It was a way of life that, by its very nature, was sustainable. People used what they had around them, and there was no mass production or excessive waste. Each item had value, and the effort put into creating these goods came with respect for the materials themselves.

But then, something monumental happened. The Industrial Revolution hit, and with it, everything changed dramatically. The once slow, natural rhythm of life was replaced by the endless hum of machines, and suddenly, the connection between people and nature began to fade.

The New Age of Chemicals

As factories began to dominate the landscape, people watched their surroundings transform almost overnight. Small, quiet towns once filled with open fields and trees gave way to towering smokestacks and brick buildings. The air, once fresh and crisp, now carried the constant hum of machinery and the thick smell of coal. Streets that had been lined with cottages and market stalls were now crisscrossed with railroads and bustling with carts hauling raw materials to fuel the factories. The horizon, which used to be dotted with the shapes of hills and forests, was now crowded with chimneys belching black smoke into the sky.

For many, this change was disorienting. The familiar rhythm of life, once dictated by the sun and the seasons, was replaced by the relentless churn of the machines. People no longer woke up to the sound of roosters crowing but to the whistle of the factory, calling them to long hours of work. The simple, natural materials that had once filled their homes, such as wooden furniture, woven baskets, and handmade tools, were now being replaced by mass-produced goods made from iron, glass, and later, synthetic materials.

This new way of life felt like progress, yet it came at a cost. The connection people once felt to the land and to nature began to fade, replaced by a growing dependency on man-made creations. At the heart of this transformation was the chemical industry. Early breakthroughs in chemistry allowed for the creation of substances that could either mimic or surpass natural materials. For instance, synthetic dyes revolutionized the textile industry. Natural dyes, while beautiful, were often inconsistent in color and difficult to produce in large quantities. With synthetic dyes, factories could now churn out fabrics with bold colors that were uniform, reliable, and available on a mass scale.

This era also saw the rise of factories, vast spaces filled with machinery designed to produce goods on an unprecedented scale. Powered by steam and later by electricity, these machines could churn out products at a rate that would have been unimaginable just decades earlier. Yet, even with this newfound power, natural resources began to show their limitations. The demand for raw materials like wood, cotton, and natural oils simply couldn't keep up with the pace of industrialization.

Synthetic alternatives became the answer. They filled the gap that nature couldn't, providing industries with the building blocks they needed to expand rapidly. One of the most significant developments was the creation of synthetic plastics. Faced with a shortage of materials like ivory and tortoiseshell, inventors turned to science in search of alternatives. In 1869, John Wesley Hyatt developed celluloid, a material that mimicked the properties of natural substances but could be produced in much larger quantities. This opened the door to the widespread use of plastics. Soon after, Leo Baekeland's invention of Bakelite in 1907 marked another key moment. As the first fully synthetic plastic, Bakelite proved to be durable and versatile, finding its way into everything from electrical insulators to household goods. It was a clear sign that the world was moving away from its reliance on natural materials.

This shift wasn't limited to plastics. The development of synthetic detergents is another example of how chemical products began to replace traditional, natural items. Soaps made from animal fats and plant oils had long been used to clean clothes, dishes, and bodies. But as chemical detergents emerged, they quickly became household staples. These products, designed for convenience and efficiency, symbolized the growing reliance on artificial goods in everyday life, a reliance that would soon dominate the modern world.

How Marketing Made Us Abandon Nature

The Industrial Revolution also transformed the way goods were marketed and sold. This era saw the rise of big marketing campaigns that made synthetic products look like the ultimate solution for a better, more modern life.

At the heart of these campaigns was a clear message: synthetic products were the future. Manufacturers recognized that the novelty and convenience of these goods had wide appeal, so they framed them as symbols of progress and sophistication. A prime example of this was the promotion of synthetic fibers like nylon. At events such as the 1939 World's Fair, DuPont proudly introduced nylon stockings in its "Wonder World of Chemistry" exhibit. The marketing emphasized their durability and shine, presenting them as superior to traditional silk. Positioning nylon as a superior choice encouraged consumers to link synthetic materials with modern living.

Companies understood the power of reaching people through new forms of media like print ads, radio, and billboards, making sure their message was heard everywhere. Companies also used radio commercials during the Great Depression to make their products household names.

What made this marketing approach so powerful was the "brain twister" effect. Companies subtly made us believe that the old, natural ways of living were outdated, inefficient, and even inferior. It was a psychological twist that convinced people to view their traditional practices as relics of the past. Synthetic fibers like nylon were hailed as superior to silk, and new cleaning products were portrayed as labor-saving miracles compared to traditional soaps.

As mass production made these synthetic products more affordable, they became accessible to more people, particularly the growing middle class. What was once considered a luxury was now within reach of everyday consumers, and this availability was framed as a symbol of modernity and success. The ads painted a picture that to truly live a better, more sophisticated life, one had to leave behind the old ways. This brain twister took hold, shaping consumer habits and pushing synthetic products into every aspect of life.

Voices of Caution

Looking back today, we wonder how so many warning signs went unnoticed. But when we dig deeper, it's clear that the allure of progress, the excitement of something new, often blinds us to the costs. During this period, as industries expanded and new products promised to make life easier, those early warnings about pollution and health risks seemed easy to brush aside.

At a time when the promise of innovation was bright, a few voices spoke out about the dark side of this rapid expansion. One of the earliest red flags came from the very heart of the revolution: the chemical industry. Factories churned out massive amounts of chemicals like sulfuric acid and soda ash, which were vital for manufacturing goods on a large scale. But alongside this production came vast amounts of industrial waste. Soda production, in particular, left behind harmful alkaline byproducts that were dumped into rivers and fields, poisoning water supplies and damaging surrounding ecosystems. The issue became so severe that it led to one of the first environmental regulations in 1863, which aimed to limit factory emissions. However, even with this legislation, the economic benefits of keeping the factories running full steam often outweighed any serious consideration for environmental consequences.

Air pollution was another growing concern. The widespread burning of coal to fuel the factories blanketed industrial cities with thick layers of smog. Cities like Manchester and London became infamous for their polluted air, which not only caused severe respiratory issues for people but also left lasting damage to plants and wildlife. Despite these visible signs of harm, the drive to keep factories humming and profits flowing kept the warnings largely ignored. Economic growth remained the priority, even as the environment and public health suffered significant damage.

Waterways, too, became casualties in the pursuit of progress. Factories often treated rivers as convenient disposal systems, dumping industrial waste such as chemicals, debris, and oils into them without a second thought. This contamination poisoned the water and harmed every form of life that depended on it. Aquatic life suffered, ecosystems began to collapse, and for the communities that relied on these rivers for drinking water, sanitation, or agriculture, the consequences were immediate and devastating. One infamous example is the Cuyahoga River in Ohio, which became a symbol of unchecked industrial pollution. The river was so heavily contaminated by oily waste that it caught fire—more than once.

Beyond the impact on water bodies, factories also required vast amounts of raw materials, leading to widespread deforestation and habitat destruction. Forests were felled, minerals were extracted, and fossil fuels were burned in unprecedented quantities. The immediate goal was to feed the growing industrial beast, with little regard for the long-term consequences. As natural resources were stripped away, ecosystems were left vulnerable, and biodiversity dwindled.

Despite these growing signs of environmental degradation, the warnings were consistently pushed aside. The promise of convenience, modernity, and economic gain continued to outweigh any concerns about sustainability or the future. And this trade-off—short-term gain at the expense of long-term well-being—is something we still wrestle with today. The choices made during this period set a precedent for the unchecked exploitation of resources, a legacy we are still grappling with as we confront the environmental crises of our time.

This journey through history goes beyond satisfying our curiosity or looking back. I hope it felt a bit like stepping into a time machine, taking us back to the dawn of the Industrial Revolution. This is just the beginning of our journey. To truly transform our present, it's essential that we keep following this historical path a bit longer. Only by fully understanding where we come from can we reshape where we're headed and work towards a more balanced, sustainable future.

Chapter 2

Globalization and the Digital Consumer Revolution

Moving forward through history, a significant change is on the horizon that will transform the way we live our daily lives all over the world. The years after the Industrial Revolution were marked by a slow but steady buildup towards what we now recognize as the era of globalization. This was a time when goods, ideas, and cultural values flowed more freely across borders, reshaping societies in ways that were once unimaginable.

For many, globalization was seen as progress, an era marked by the vast movement of products and the promise of modern conveniences. But beneath the surface, it also carried with it a subtle but steady replacement of traditional practices with industrialized consumer patterns. In developing countries like India, this transformation became particularly evident.

This change didn't happen overnight. It began with the presence of global corporations, enticing the population with promises of convenience. Daily-use goods were among the first to capture attention. Synthetic cleaning products, for instance, were introduced as modern alternatives that promised to simplify household chores. The appeal was clear: busy urban lifestyles could benefit from the quick solutions these products offered, sparking a curiosity to try the "new" in place of what had been done for generations.

In stores that once displayed locally made soaps and natural cleaning powders, shelves began to fill with brightly packaged detergents, hand washes, and other chemically infused items, all claiming to be easier, faster, and more effective.

In the cosmetics industry, this shift was stark. I remember a time, not too long ago, when the everyday rituals of life felt much more grounded in nature. Beauty routines, for instance, were simple yet deeply meaningful. In many Indian households, women used turmeric, sandalwood, and neem—natural ingredients that had been passed down through generations. Back then, synthetic products were not entirely absent from Indian markets, but they hadn't yet taken over. The scale of their presence was far smaller, and their influence was not as overpowering.

Yet, as global brands entered the Indian market, they brought with them an entirely different narrative. Do you remember the first time you saw those glossy ads? Synthetic cosmetics were showcased as miracles in bottles—instant fixes, promising flawless beauty. These ads made you feel like using them was a way to be part of something bigger, something modern and sophisticated, as if natural beauty wasn't enough anymore.

But it wasn't just the beauty industry that changed. The food we ate began to shift as well. Do you remember how meals used to be? Freshly prepared, locally sourced, and shared around a family table? Globalization brought fast-food giants into our cities and, with them, a new way of thinking about food. Quick, processed, and packed with artificial additives, these meals were designed for convenience rather than nourishment. The idea of grabbing a burger or a slice of pizza felt like an exciting, modern way to eat, but with that shift came a growing dependence on processed foods.

Trade-Offs of Globalization

Looking back, it's striking to see how deeply these changes have taken root in our everyday lives. And while the allure of synthetic products promised ease and modernity, it's worth asking—what have we lost in this shift? What have we left behind in our rush to embrace the global and the new?

There was a darker side to this massive shift that impacted the environment and even our health. One of the most glaring examples is the explosion of synthetic materials, especially plastics. Think about it: almost everything we buy comes wrapped in plastic. It's everywhere, from packaging to everyday household items. But unlike the traditional materials our ancestors used, plastics don't just disappear. They linger for centuries, choking landfills, clogging oceans, and polluting our environment in ways we never fully anticipated. The convenience that synthetic materials offered quickly turned into a nightmare of waste management.

But the impact of globalization doesn't end there. Along with it came the powerful influence of multinational corporations (MNCs), whose operations spread deep into countries like India. One of the major impacts of these MNCs is what's often called "pollution havens." In simpler terms, these corporations set up factories in countries where environmental regulations are weaker and where the rules are more lenient, allowing them to dump waste and emit pollutants. And who bears the cost of this? Developing nations like ours face the costs of the air we breathe, the water we drink, and the land we live on.

Take, for example, the continued use of harmful pesticides in developing countries, which are chemicals banned in many wealthier nations. These toxic substances, outlawed in the very countries that produce them, are still being sprayed over fields in regions where regulations are weaker. The consequences for local communities are devastating. In Central America, banana plantations operated by companies have relied on insecticides so harmful that they've caused infertility among workers. These are real lives, real families, directly harmed because cutting costs was prioritized over health and safety.

Resource exploitation is another painful chapter in this story. The relentless demand for raw materials, driven by global markets, has led to reckless extraction practices that have left landscapes scarred and ecosystems disrupted. Here in India, mining operations, fueled by global demand, have caused widespread deforestation, soil erosion, and water contamination. The effects impact the environment and traditional livelihoods that have existed in harmony with nature for centuries.

If we consider how these corporations shape our desires and behaviors, the picture becomes even more troubling. Through relentless marketing and advertising, they've ingrained in us a craving for newness, convenience, and instant results. Television, social media, and billboards constantly push us toward a lifestyle of continuous consumption, where synthetic products are equated with success, modernity, and progress.

The Consumerism Engine

As if globalization hadn't already pushed us deep enough into a culture of consumerism, the digital age accelerated this shift in ways unimaginable just a few decades ago. With the rise of the internet, smartphones, and social media, products were no longer just sold to us through billboards or television ads. Now, they followed us everywhere: on every website, in every app, and through every screen we scrolled. And as you might guess, the products pushed at us weren't those made from time-tested, natural ingredients or rooted in sustainable practices. They were synthetics, marketed for their "efficiency," "modern appeal," and, of course, convenience.

One of the main driving forces behind this digital transformation is personalized advertising. Algorithms have come to know us intimately, including our browsing habits, social media posts, and the products we pause to look at. Platforms like Facebook, Instagram, and Google collect this data to tailor ads that closely align with our tastes. Ever noticed how one search for a moisturizer suddenly leads to a flood of ads for cosmetics and skincare items across all your devices? That's no coincidence. These algorithms are specifically designed to capture our attention, increasing the chances that we'll buy items we may not have even considered before. And because they're so good at targeting our specific desires, we're often drawn toward synthetic options, influenced by digital ads that make them look essential to our lives.

Also, it is impossible to talk about the digital age without acknowledging the profound influence of platforms like Instagram and YouTube. These spaces have completely transformed how we discover and engage with products, particularly synthetic ones. At the forefront of this transformation are influencers whose curated lives have become a key part of modern marketing.

The power of influencers lies in their relatability. Unlike traditional advertisements, where the distance between the brand and the consumer is stark, influencers bridge that gap. They invite us into their lives, sharing what feels like personal, behind-the-scenes glimpses of their daily habits. But what happens when these glimpses are filled with endorsements for synthetic products? Take, for instance, an influencer showcasing their morning skincare routine. It might involve a series of chemical-laden beauty products, all presented as part of their flawless complexion. Because we trust them, it's easy to get swept into thinking that these products are desirable and necessary.

In this way, influencers and celebrities have effectively become walking, talking billboards. The products they promote, often synthetic, become associated with success, beauty, and modern living. And because these platforms are visual and fast-paced, the products are embedded into the content we consume daily, normalizing their use without much thought.

It's not just influencers who've shifted our focus toward synthetic products; celebrities with massive followings add another layer to this trend. When a well-known figure endorses a product, it carries a certain weight, an unspoken validation that this item must be worth trying. Their reach and influence extend far beyond any traditional ad, making consumers feel as though they, too, can attain a piece of that celebrity's success or beauty by simply purchasing the endorsed item.

Imagine a celebrity promoting a hair care product on Instagram, suggesting it's the key to their hair care routine. Or a beauty icon sharing their "must-have" skincare routine filled with products containing synthetic chemicals. Without even realizing it, we start viewing these synthetic products as shortcuts to the lifestyle they represent, often sidelining traditional practices that value sustainability and natural ingredients.

This cycle of influence has essentially become a consumerism engine. We're constantly presented with new synthetic "must-haves," while these platforms and celebrities fuel a demand that seems endless. And in this setup, we start to feel less like individuals and more like cogs in a giant machine, driven to consume without pause.

What we see here is the complete opposite of the philosophy of rooted living, where the body and the world around us are viewed with reverence and care. Instead, this system encourages a detachment from both. It's about quantity over quality and speed over mindfulness, which is a far cry from the balanced, natural way of living we strive to return to.

The Early Signs of Change

Yet, there's a silver lining in this digital era that's hard to overlook. The same digital age that's been responsible for promoting endless consumerism and synthetic lifestyles is also giving rise to something quite hopeful: a counter-narrative.

The digital age has brought with it a wave of awareness. People are beginning to see through the consumerism engine, questioning the choices they've been led to make. It's almost as though, in recognizing how far we've strayed from natural living, we've realized we might be approaching a point of no return. Thankfully, this recognition has sparked a growing movement towards natural and sustainable living—a fortunate outcome of this digitally connected world.

One of the most powerful tools the digital age has given us is access to information. We now have the ability to research, read testimonials, and explore the science behind the products we use daily. We can fact-check, dive into research, and uncover the truth behind flashy marketing claims. This kind of access allows us to look beyond the surface and question what we're being sold. It exposes us to things like greenwashing, where companies make false claims about the sustainability of their products just to capitalize on the trend. And with this knowledge, many are making more informed choices, leaning towards natural and herbal alternatives that truly align with their values.

These digital platforms have also created spaces where personal stories about alternative lifestyles, like sustainable and rooted living, are shared. Many of these stories paint a compelling picture of the benefits of minimizing synthetic products and seeking harmony with nature. But as inspiring as some of these stories are, the reality is often more complicated. A disappointing number of them misunderstand what sustainable or rooted living truly means. These terms have become buzzwords, thrown around without depth, reducing a profound way of life to a trend. People are eager to embrace this lifestyle, but they often feel lost and lack the deeper understanding and guidance needed to make meaningful changes.

Even when some genuinely try to live this way, they end up feeling overwhelmed, unsure of where to start or how to stay consistent. The complexity of the change, which involves tackling misleading product labels and rethinking their entire approach to daily living, can be exhausting. For many, it feels like an unattainable ideal, leaving them disillusioned and disconnected from the very essence of rooted living.

That's where the pages ahead will prove helpful. Together, we'll start with the "why." This is what I call an awakening. It's the process of peeling back the layers, becoming aware of the dangers hidden in our everyday choices, and realizing how far we've drifted from the natural balance that sustains us. This awakening is about making sense of what's really happening. Once we're clear on the risks and understand why this change is so crucial, the "how" will follow naturally.

Chapter 3

The Awakening – Realizing the Hazards of Chemical Products

Let's take a moment to reflect on something Albert Einstein once said: "The world as we have created it is a process of our thinking. It cannot be changed without changing our thinking." This insight challenges us to rethink the concept of sustainability, a term that has evolved over time but often strays from its original meaning. In many contexts today, it's used as a buzzword rather than a genuine commitment. True sustainability goes beyond reducing harm; it creates harmony between humanity and the environment. Let's explore what that really means. Those words remind us that any real change begins in the mind. And when we talk about awakening, it transforms how we think, especially regarding chemicals and their place in our world.

As we begin this awakening, an important question needs to be asked: *What's the single element that connects you to the world around you?*

It's your body. This sacred vessel links you to nature, the very space we cherish and often refer to as divine. So, if we are to awaken to the realities of our chemical-filled world, it has to start with our bodies and how we interact with the natural world.

Are we binding our bodies to nature in a harmonious, balanced way? Unfortunately, the truth is far from that. Today, it's the intrusive ties of chemicals that bind our bodies to the environment. Let me explain what that means. Think about your everyday routine—the products you use without a second thought. You start your morning by washing your face with a refreshing face wash, step into the shower and lather up with a fragrant body cleanser, massaging shampoo into your hair. Afterward, there's deodorant, moisturizer, and maybe some makeup before heading out into the world. Does this sound familiar? Well, I've been there, so I understand. Each of those products, however, holds a hidden truth. They're packed with a mix of chemicals formulated to clean, protect, and improve their appeal.

But here's something we don't often think about: Have you ever stopped to ask yourself what kind of impact these everyday products have on the environment?

The Environmental Toll of Chemicals

The products we use every day might seem harmless on the surface, but their journey begins long before they reach your bathroom shelf. Behind the scenes, the process of creating these products involves extracting and synthesizing various chemicals, many of which come from petroleum. This is where the environmental toll starts.

The production of synthetic ingredients demands a significant amount of energy, much of it coming from non-renewable resources. Petroleum, for instance, is the base for many synthetic components in everyday items like shampoos, lotions, and cosmetics. But the process of extracting and refining petroleum is far from harmless—it's a heavy burden on the planet.

The very act of oil and gas exploration often takes place in some of the world's most ecologically sensitive regions, such as the Arctic or the

Congo Basin. These operations disrupt fragile ecosystems, interfere with wildlife migrations, and contribute to biodiversity loss. Drilling for oil may provide the ingredients for our personal care products, but it leaves behind a trail of destruction that we can't ignore. One catastrophic example is the BP Deepwater Horizon oil spill in 2010, which left a devastating mark on marine life. The spill contaminated thousands of square miles of sea surface, killing vast numbers of seabirds, marine mammals, and sea turtles.

The strain on natural resources doesn't stop with petroleum; water plays an equally significant role in the production of personal care products. Manufacturing these items requires enormous quantities of water at various stages—mixing ingredients, cooling machinery, and cleaning equipment between batches. Factories often use Clean-in-Place (CIP) systems to sanitize their machines, but these processes consume vast amounts of both water and energy. In areas already grappling with water scarcity, this intensive use further strains local water supplies, increasing environmental stress.

What makes this even more concerning is the waste that follows. After being used in production, the wastewater—often laden with chemical residues—flows into rivers and oceans, typically without proper treatment. This threatens aquatic ecosystems and risks contaminating water sources that communities rely on for drinking and agriculture. Water, an essential resource for life, becomes a conduit for pollution, harming both the environment and people.

Beyond water, another hidden cost of producing synthetic personal care products lies in the minerals and metals used for ingredients. Take mica, for example, the mineral responsible for giving cosmetics their shimmering glow. Mined extensively, often in fragile ecosystems, mica extraction can lead to deforestation, soil erosion, and water contamination as runoff from mining operations seeps into nearby water bodies. The consequences of this are far-reaching: not only is the environment left scarred, but the communities that rely on these ecosystems suffer as well. Similarly, the demand for other minerals needed for pigments and preservatives continues to deplete natural reserves, creating a cycle of environmental degradation.

Beyond the water usage and mineral depletion, the afterlife of these products creates a new set of challenges. Once these products are rinsed off in the shower, the chemicals don't just disappear. When washed down the drain, these chemicals make their way into waterways, bringing with them serious consequences for aquatic life. Think about microbeads—those tiny plastic particles used in face scrubs. They pass right through water treatment systems and end up in rivers and oceans. Marine animals often mistake them for food, and when ingested, these microplastics can cause internal harm or even death. Then there's triclosan, a common antibacterial agent in soaps and toothpaste. It disrupts hormone functions in aquatic species, affecting their ability to reproduce and grow, which, in turn, throws entire ecosystems out of balance.

Soil also pays the price. When wastewater sludge containing these chemicals is used as fertilizer or dumped in landfills, compounds like parabens and phthalates seep into the ground. These substances alter the microbial communities vital to healthy, fertile soil. Over time, this degradation can harm agricultural productivity, threatening not only the environment but also food security.

Often overlooked, air pollution from personal care products is another serious concern. The aerosol sprays we use release VOCs that worsen air quality and contribute to climate change. Add to that the carbon dioxide emissions from the production of certain ingredients, and you can see how these everyday products have a far-reaching environmental impact.

As we take a closer look at the air we breathe, we notice another silent culprit that adds to the problem: the packaging of chemical products. While we often focus on the products inside, the packaging itself carries a heavy environmental burden. Think about the sheer amount of plastic packaging wrapped around our shampoos, lotions, and cosmetics. The beauty industry alone is responsible for producing over 120 billion units of packaging every year. That's a staggering amount of waste, most of it in the form of plastic.

Plastic is a go-to material for the beauty industry because it's cheap, durable, and convenient. But here's the issue: it comes from petroleum, a non-renewable resource that requires extensive energy to extract and refine. The process contributes to environmental degradation at every step, and once we've used that bottle or container, it's typically discarded. Most of this plastic ends up in landfills, oceans, or incinerators because cosmetic packaging is rarely recyclable. Greenpeace USA reports that only a tiny fraction of plastics used in packaging are recyclable, and most cosmetic containers aren't made from these more recyclable types.

What happens next is concerning. This discarded plastic lingers in the environment for centuries, taking up to 450 years to decompose. In that time, it can release harmful chemicals into the soil and water, impacting ecosystems and potentially making its way back to us through the food chain. Wildlife is also affected, with many animals ingesting or becoming trapped in plastic debris.

It's hard to overlook the fact that the packaging, designed for convenience, becomes an enduring problem for the environment. I understand that this is a lot to take in, but grasping these consequences is a crucial step in rethinking the products we use and their impact on the world around us.

Health Impacts of Chemical Exposure

The effects of chemical products on the environment are deeply concerning, but the truth is, they're doing just as much harm to us. The products we use every day, shampoos, lotions, deodorants, and cosmetics, come with a hidden cost. While they might promise to make us feel clean, fresh, and beautiful, they also expose us to chemicals that can slowly wreak havoc on our health.

When you think about it, everything you apply to your skin, spray in the air, or wash your hair with has to go somewhere. Much of it is absorbed by your body or inhaled into your lungs. Over time, prolonged exposure to these chemicals can lead to a range of health problems. And sadly, many of us are unaware of the toll these everyday products can take.

One of the most overlooked effects of using chemical-laden products is how they can affect our ability to breathe. Have you ever sprayed a mist of deodorant or hair spray and felt a tickle in your throat or a sudden urge to cough? That's because many of these products contain volatile organic compounds (VOCs) and synthetic fragrances that release harmful particles into the air. Every time you use them, you're breathing those chemicals in.

For those with respiratory conditions like asthma or COPD, this can be especially dangerous. These chemicals can worsen breathing difficulties, triggering symptoms like wheezing, shortness of breath, or even more severe asthma attacks. Studies have found that people who regularly use cleaning products or cosmetics with high levels of VOCs are at increased risk of developing chronic respiratory problems over time. It's something we all need to be more aware of as we fill our homes and bathrooms with products that pollute the very air we breathe.

Then there's the issue of skin allergies. Many of the chemicals used to make personal care products smell good, last longer, or look a certain way can irritate our skin, sometimes severely. Fragrances, preservatives, and dyes are among the most common culprits. You might notice an itchy red rash after using a new lotion, or hives after switching to a different brand of shampoo. These are signs that your body is reacting to an allergen in the product.

Over time, continuous exposure can lead to conditions like contact dermatitis, where the skin becomes inflamed, itchy, and painful. It's your body's way of saying, "Enough is enough." Allergic reactions to chemicals in personal care products can sometimes be so severe that they cause long-term skin sensitivity, making it difficult for people to find products they can safely use.

There's an even more concerning issue that many people aren't fully aware of: the long-term, systemic impact of chemicals used in personal care products. It's not just about what happens on the surface of our skin or in our lungs, but what goes on deeper inside our bodies over time.

Take phthalates, for example. These chemicals are found in a variety of cosmetics and personal care items, where they help products retain their fragrance and texture. However, phthalates are endocrine-disrupting chemicals (EDCs), meaning they can interfere with our hormonal system. Research has linked them to reproductive health issues, developmental problems, and even complications during pregnancy.

Another group of chemicals that has raised significant concerns are parabens, which are often used as preservatives in products like lotions, shampoos, and makeup. While parabens help prevent mold and bacteria growth, studies suggest they may also contribute to hormone disruption, which can increase the risk of certain cancers. Though they might seem harmless in small doses, the problem lies in the daily, repeated use of multiple products containing these chemicals.

Additionally, ingredients like titanium dioxide (TiO2), commonly found in sunscreens and cosmetics, are also under scrutiny. Though generally considered safe, the concern arises with the nanoparticles of TiO2, which under certain conditions can penetrate the skin. Once absorbed, they can potentially cause oxidative stress and damage cells.

Over time, these daily exposures accumulate, putting our bodies under a continuous chemical load. For example, ongoing exposure to endocrine-disrupting chemicals in personal care products has been linked in some studies to broader health issues, including an increased risk of metabolic disorders like obesity and diabetes. These aren't conditions we can dismiss—they affect our quality of life, our long-term health, and even the health of future generations.

The cumulative impact of this daily chemical exposure emphasizes why it's so important to become aware of what we're putting on our bodies. We can't ignore the potential harm caused by products we've grown so accustomed to using. Understanding the risks associated with long-term exposure is a key part of waking up to the reality of the chemical ties that bind us.

Breaking the Cycle of Demand

After realizing the toll that chemical products take on our bodies and the environment, you may feel a strong urge to act. But here's where doubt often creeps in: *Does my decision alone make any real difference?* It's a valid question, one that many of us ask. First, let's remember that even on a personal level, choosing to step away from chemical-based products directly protects you, reducing your own exposure to substances that carry long-term health risks. But beyond that, your choice goes further than you might imagine.

Imagine if everyone hesitated, thinking that one individual's actions wouldn't matter. Change would never take root. However, when each of us makes a small, intentional choice to distance ourselves from these products, it can lead to a meaningful impact. Think about it this way: every purchase you make, or don't make, sends a message to the companies behind these products. When more people choose products that are safe, sustainable, and chemical-free, it signals a shift in demand. Companies will eventually have no choice but to notice.

In fact, studies show that informed consumers often avoid products with harmful chemicals once they're aware of the risks. And it's this awareness that drives market demand. When enough people start to opt-out of purchasing chemical-laden products, production slows down. With less demand, there's less incentive for companies to extract and refine the non-renewable resources needed for these products. This, in turn, leads to fewer pollutants, less plastic waste, and a reduction in environmental harm.

Take shampoos containing sulfates or parabens, for example. If a large portion of consumers choose to avoid these ingredients, manufacturers will have no choice but to cut back on their production. With that reduction, we start seeing real environmental benefits such as less chemical runoff polluting our water systems, fewer emissions from manufacturing plants, and a drop in plastic waste from packaging that often ends up in landfills or our oceans.

Consumer choices also play a critical role in shaping corporate behavior. Companies, always eager to meet market demand, are increasingly responding to the call for safer and more sustainable products. This is why we've seen a rise in brands that emphasize environmentally friendly practices, opting for biodegradable materials and committing to reducing waste. As more people lean toward buying from these companies, the pressure on others to adopt more sustainable business models grows.

What's even more encouraging is how consumer behavior can push for real change at the policy level. When enough people advocate for safer products, regulatory bodies often follow suit, enforcing stricter guidelines on chemical usage. We've already seen this happen with phthalates, as an outcry from informed consumers led to regulations that restricted their use in various products.

This pattern of consumer-driven change isn't unique to phthalates. In fact, it's part of a broader trend where individual choices, when multiplied, influence entire industries. Let's look at two additional examples: the rise of organic food and the reduction in plastic bag usage. The organic food movement is one of the most striking examples of how people, driven by health and environmental concerns, can reshape industries. Over the past few decades, more and more individuals have turned to organic products, fueled by a growing awareness of the potential health risks associated with pesticides and synthetic fertilizers used in conventional farming. This became a powerful movement that transformed the food industry globally. To give you an idea, since 2000, sales of organic food have skyrocketed by over $100 billion, with North America leading the way in this shift.

What's fascinating is that this demand didn't just affect what's available on supermarket shelves. It actually led to a massive change in how food is grown. Organic farming practices—those that avoid synthetic chemicals and focus on maintaining ecological balance—moved from niche to mainstream. Countries like Australia, Argentina, and China have now dedicated huge portions of land to organic farming, reflecting a deeper societal shift towards health-conscious and sustainable living.

Another powerful example of how individual actions can create real change is the global reduction in plastic bag usage. This shift has been largely driven by a combination of consumer behavior and policy changes. In many places, public awareness campaigns and government regulations have worked together to drastically cut down on single-use plastic bags, which have been a major source of environmental harm.

In 2016, India introduced a nationwide ban on plastic bags in several states, with Maharashtra leading the charge by enforcing strict penalties for plastic bag usage. This movement was further supported by various retailers and local initiatives that encouraged the use of reusable alternatives.

In places like Delhi and Bengaluru, the combined efforts of government enforcement and public participation saw a significant drop in single-use plastic bags. Several large retail chains in India began offering reusable bags to customers and even charged a small fee for plastic ones, pushing consumers toward more sustainable choices. Initiatives like the "Swachh Bharat Abhiyan" (Clean India Mission) also played a key role in raising public awareness about the harmful effects of plastic pollution on the environment.

While plastic bags haven't been completely eliminated, there has been a widespread decline in their usage across cities and towns. Shoppers are increasingly bringing their own reusable bags, and the sight of plastic bags littering the streets has visibly diminished in many areas. This shift in consumer behavior highlights the power of awareness and collective action.

This example of plastic bags shows us a clear path forward when it comes to reducing our reliance on chemical-based products. Just as public awareness helped shift behavior in the case of plastic, we can raise awareness about the harmful impacts of chemicals in personal care products. If enough of us make conscious choices to avoid these products, it will force manufacturers to rethink their practices and adopt more sustainable alternatives.

These examples highlight a crucial part of the "why" behind our choices: our individual actions and decisions matter deeply, directly influencing the natural world around us. However, there is more to uncover, something fundamental that nature itself teaches us through its design.

Understanding this natural cycle reveals what's at stake when we step away from conscious, thoughtful decisions. It shows us the importance of aligning our actions with nature's design by choosing to reduce waste, regenerate resources, and respect the finite systems that sustain us.

When we fail to act with intention, we disrupt these cycles and risk harm to both our planet and future generations. This perspective reminds us why every choice matters. It extends to what we nurture, creating an ecosystem of thoughtful consumption that reflects the wisdom of nature itself.

Chapter 4

The Circular Economy – Rediscovering Simplicity in a Complex World

In nature, nothing goes to waste.

When a leaf falls, it doesn't stay on the ground for long. It breaks down into the soil, feeding the tree it came from. Birds collect twigs to build nests, reusing what's already there. Even a tiny flower, when it withers, gives back to the earth, nourishing new life. Every part has a role, working together in an endless, natural cycle.

Now think of your street. A plastic bottle rolls along the pavement, pushed around by footsteps. Wrappers pile up in bins, spilling over onto the ground. Water struggles to flow through drains clogged with rubbish. These items don't disappear or return to a cycle. They stay where they are, piling up, with nowhere to go.

This difference between nature and the city shows two ways of living. One is circular, where everything is reused and renewed. The other is linear, where things are taken, used, and thrown away without considering what happens next. For too long, we've chosen the second path, creating more waste and losing valuable resources.

But what if we followed nature's way?

What if, like nature, we could design our lives to reduce waste, regenerate resources, and create cycles that work—not against the environment but with it? This is the idea behind the circular economy—a system that isn't only about recycling but about rethinking how we use everything, from the smallest objects in our homes to the biggest systems that shape our lives.

This system of reuse and renewal offers a blueprint for how we could rethink our own lives following our awakening and the systems we depend on.

Understanding the Circular Economy

Think of the everyday things we use, from the water bottle you grab on a hot day to the plastic-wrapped snacks that line your kitchen shelves. Each one starts somewhere crafted in a factory, shaped by machines, and delivered to us with the promise of convenience.

But what happens after we're done with them? Most of these items follow the same path: used once, tossed aside, and forgotten. This "take, make, dispose" model has become so normal that we rarely pause to question it.

Take a single plastic bottle, for example. It begins its life deep beneath the earth, where crude oil is extracted and transported to factories, its transformation powered by energy-intensive machines. The air around these plants smells sharp and metallic, a reminder of the processes needed to shape that oil into the smooth, clear bottle you hold in your hand. Once formed, it's filled, capped, and wrapped in vibrant branding designed to catch your eye on a store shelf.

You buy it on a sweltering afternoon, its cool surface beading with condensation as you twist off the cap. The water inside quenches your thirst quickly, and without a second thought, you toss the empty bottle away. Maybe it lands in a dustbin or a recycling bag. Or perhaps, like so many others, it's dropped on the pavement, forgotten in the rush of daily life.

But this is only the beginning of its story. In the best-case scenario, the bottle might be transported to a recycling facility, but often, it doesn't make it there. Instead, it's carted to a landfill, buried under mounds of waste where it will sit for centuries, breaking down into smaller and smaller pieces but never fully disappearing.

Sometimes, the journey takes a darker turn. Caught by a gust of wind, it tumbles into a nearby drain, carried by rainwater to a river. The current pulls it along, bobbing and spinning with other debris, until it reaches the ocean. Here, it drifts into one of the planet's mmassive garbage patches, swirling gyres of waste that stretch for miles. Beneath the waves, sunlight and saltwater break the bottle into microplastics—tiny fragments invisible to the eye but impossible to remove.

These fragments enter the marine food chain. Fish mistake them for food, their stomachs filling with plastic instead of nourishment. Coral reefs, already fragile, are suffocated by the chemicals leaching from these plastics. Sea turtles choke on larger pieces, mistaking them for jellyfish, while seabirds carry the debris back to their nests, unknowingly feeding their chicks fragments of waste. The impact affects not only marine life but also the humans who rely on the ocean for food and livelihoods. Every microplastic ingested by a fish becomes part of the cycle that eventually leads back to us.

This single bottle, so light and disposable in your hand, leaves a trail of destruction long after its brief moment of use. And this is just a small example of where it all begins —a reminder of the straight-line systems we've built that prioritize quick solutions over lasting ones.

Now, think of a glass bottle instead. It's heavier, more solid. You finish what's inside, clean it, and send it back to be refilled. If it chips or breaks, it can be melted and reshaped into something new. This bottle doesn't follow the same linear path. It fits into a cycle, one designed to reuse, regenerate, and reduce waste. This is the essence of the circular economy: finding ways to keep resources in motion, creating systems where nothing is wasted and everything has a purpose.

The circular economy isn't a far-off concept or a policy discussion—it's something we can start right now in our homes and communities. It's about fixing the things we'd normally throw away, choosing items that last, and rethinking what we truly need. Every time you refill a bottle, mend a cracked clay pot, or buy something built to last, you're part of this shift.

A report by the Ellen MacArthur Foundation in 2023 revealed the staggering potential of this approach. Transitioning to a circular economy could cut global greenhouse gas emissions by 45%. Imagine a world where waste isn't a problem to solve because everything has a place in a cycle—a world that regenerates rather than depletes.

This is not a way of living that reduces waste, but a way that aligns with how nature has worked for millions of years. It's a way of living that values what we have, looks to the future, and embraces a natural rhythm of renewal and regeneration.

The Original Circular Economy: Nature

When you peel a piece of fruit or toss vegetable scraps into the bin, it's easy to think of it as waste. But in nature, there's no such thing. What we see as leftovers becomes nourishment for the next cycle. Leaves fall, roots absorb nutrients, and new growth begins again. Each part is connected, creating a cycle that regenerates life over and over. It's a quiet process, but it keeps the world moving in balance.

Now think about how we handle things in our own lives. A broken chair, a torn shirt, or even a jar once emptied—it's often easier to throw them away than to imagine how they could fit back into the system. Yet, every item we discard lingers somewhere, refusing to fade like leaves in a forest or scraps in the soil. These choices create breaks in the cycle, leaving behind piles of waste that don't belong in the natural flow.

Nature's way isn't complicated. It shows us that nothing has to be useless. The energy and matter in one form transform into something else, making every piece valuable. This focuses on more than composting or reusing items—it's a mindset that values connection, where every choice has a purpose.

Think about what you've read in the earlier chapters. From reusing glass jars to growing fresh herbs at home, each small habit reflects this natural cycle. Even simple choices, like cooking with durable cookware or selecting biodegradable products, reflect this way of living—one that respects what we use and how it returns to the earth.

Take composting as an example. It's not a new idea but one that turns scraps into rich soil, reducing the need for chemical fertilizers while feeding plants that grow our food. Research from the Indian Ministry of Environment (2022) shows that composting organic waste can cut landfill contributions by 30%, reducing methane emissions and giving back to the soil in the process. This is nature's cycle in action, showing how even the smallest choices can create meaningful change.

It's the same with choosing items that last. Remember the stainless-steel tiffin boxes that have been in our homes for as long as we can recall? Or how our elders used to do things with sustainability in mind? A bamboo toothbrush doesn't need frequent replacement; it becomes a part of your routine, showing care for both yourself and the world around you. These decisions might seem small, but they mirror the way nature works: simple, thoughtful, and connected.

Living this way doesn't mean dramatic changes or giving up convenience—it's making choices that feel aligned with something deeper. It's seeing the value in what we already have and finding ways to keep things moving, regenerating, and renewing. Nature has been doing this forever. It's up to us to remember how to follow its lead.

Let's explore how.

Practical Steps to Embrace Circular Living

It starts small, with the things you already have at home. Look around your kitchen, your cupboards, or your storeroom. That empty pickle jar doesn't need to be thrown away—it could store spices or grains. The torn cotton saree tucked away in a corner could become soft cleaning cloths. By repurposing what we have, we extend the life of everyday items, reducing waste and finding new value in things we might have overlooked.

Think about leftovers—not just food but scraps like vegetable peels or the water you used to rinse rice. Instead of discarding them, they can nurture your garden. Vegetable scraps can go into a compost bin, and that rice water? It's a simple, natural fertilizer that plants love. Even in a small flat or balcony, composting can be an easy and rewarding way to create something useful from waste. Kitchen scraps break down over time, turning into rich, nutrient-packed soil for your plants.

Switching from single-use plastics to durable alternatives is another way to make a big difference. Stainless steel or glass water bottles can replace disposable plastic ones. Beeswax wraps are a natural, reusable alternative to cling film, perfect for covering bowls or wrapping food. Instead of piling up with throwaway shopping bags, sturdy cloth bags—ones you can fold into a corner of your purse or backpack—make grocery runs easier and more sustainable. It's not about overhauling everything overnight but replacing one disposable item at a time with something built to last.

Supporting brands and businesses that are part of this movement helps grow the idea of circular living beyond your home, encouraging industries to think sustainably too.

Benefits of Circular Living

Making these small shifts transforms more than your home—it reshapes how you connect with the world around you. Circular living involves reducing waste; it's a way to create balance, improve your health, and nurture deeper connections within your community.. The benefits are far-reaching, yet they start with simple choices.

When you switch to biodegradable and non-toxic products, you're protecting not just the environment but your own well-being. Wooden cooking tools, bamboo brushes, or natural cleaning solutions create cleaner, safer spaces. Washing vegetables feels different when you know the detergent in the sink is gentle on both your hands and the planet. Storing food in glass jars instead of plastic feels lighter, knowing it avoids leaching harmful chemicals. Each change adds to a sense of ease and peace, building a home where every decision feels intentional and aligned with care.

Repairing and reusing aren't only practical—they carry a sense of satisfaction. Fixing a favorite pair of shoes or restoring a chipped pot adds life to objects that have already served you well. Investing in durable items, like a steel tiffin box or a glass water bottle, saves money in the long run. These pieces stay with you, becoming part of your story. A well-kept cast iron pan tells of countless meals shared, while a repaired chair speaks to the thoughtfulness of choosing preservation over waste.

Beyond the walls of your home, these changes extend outward. Every product repaired or reused means fewer natural resources extracted. Mining for metals slows; forests are left standing; water systems remain unpolluted. Cleaner soil grows better crops, healthier rivers sustain more life, and unpolluted air supports thriving ecosystems. These aren't distant impacts—they're part of the same systems that provide for us daily. When resources are used wisely, they nourish everything they touch.

This way of living strengthens communities. A visit to a farmers' market becomes more than shopping; it's a moment to connect with those who grow your food, reducing the miles it travels and keeping the land healthier. Repair shops and composting drives are places to exchange not only tools but stories, creating bonds built on shared values. These spaces bring neighbors together, fostering connections that go beyond the transactional.

As these efforts grow, they create meaningful opportunities for work. Repairing, recycling, and crafting durable products provide jobs rooted in sustainability. Supporting these practices encourages industries to focus on long-term value rather than short-term gain. It's a shift that benefits everyone—workers, consumers, and the environment.

Every step you take toward circular living—whether replacing disposable items, choosing natural materials, or joining a community initiative—adds value to your life and the world around you. These choices connect us to something deeper, reminding us that care for ourselves, others, and the earth are all part of the same cycle. Circular living isn't a matter of sacrifice; it's recognizing the abundance that comes from living thoughtfully, making every action part of a system that nourishes life.

Our lives are shaped by the choices we make, both big and small. Each action—repairing something instead of discarding it, reusing items in creative ways, or picking materials that last—is part of a story larger than ourselves.

Living in alignment with the natural world isn't chasing perfection or adhering to rigid rules. It's thoughtfulness—choosing to see the potential in what we already have, finding joy in the simplicity of living lighter, and making decisions that respect the resources we share. A cracked pot isn't a problem to be solved; it's an opportunity to create something new. An old jar isn't disposable; it's a vessel for both practical use and meaningful intent.

As we welcome these small shifts, something significant begins to happen. Leftover peels and scraps turn into rich compost that nurtures soil, which, in turn, supports the food that sustains us. Durable tools, passed down through generations, become part of family meals and memories. These actions reflect care, resourcefulness, and a connection to something timeless.

Circular living doesn't mean giving something up—it's finding balance. It's stepping into a rhythm that has existed in nature for millions of years and understanding our place within it. When we approach our choices with care, we create harmony, not waste. And in doing so, we give back to the world that gives so much to us.

The systems we rely on can reflect these values, too—where waste is no longer an issue because every piece has purpose, where resources are used wisely, and where renewal is at the very centre of how we live.

This entails rediscovering balance. It means stepping into a flow that nature has followed for millions of years and recognizing our place within it. When we make choices with intention, we create harmony instead of waste. In this harmony, we find renewal, where resources are cherished, and every piece serves a purpose.

This idea of balance goes beyond just nature's design—it's about the forces that shape life itself. The next chapter will explore this deeper aspect of the "why," diving into the interplay of order and chaos in the world around us. Nature thrives not only through its circular cycles but also through the dynamic balance of these forces. Understanding this interplay helps us see how our actions, even the smallest ones, can restore harmony in a world that often feels disconnected.

Chapter 5

Entropy in Our Ecosystems – Embracing Order in Disorder

In our universe, everything around us is shaped by a constant tug-of-war between order and disorder. This balance is a natural part of life, and there's a scientific term for it that you might remember from school—entropy. It may sound like a technical word, but its impact is something we experience every day, and it holds deep meaning for how we understand our relationship with the world around us.

Entropy is a way to measure how much disorder exists in any system. To put it simply, it shows how everything, over time, tends to move from a state of order to disorder. It's tied to the second law of thermodynamics, which essentially tells us that in an isolated system, the disorder will naturally increase unless there's energy added to keep things in check. So, things fall apart, scatter, or break down unless an effort is made to keep them together.

You've probably witnessed entropy in action without even realizing it. Think about an ice cube. When it's frozen, the water molecules inside are arranged neatly and locked in place in a crystalline structure, creating a state of order. But as the ice begins to melt, those molecules start to move freely, and the structure breaks down, turning into water. What you're seeing is the increase of entropy, the move toward disorder, as the ice cube becomes part of its warmer surroundings. And once it's melted, there's no going back. That's entropy in motion.

Arthur Eddington, an astronomer and physicist, once said, "The law that entropy always increases holds, I think, the supreme position among the laws of Nature." These words stick with me because they capture the universal truth of entropy, underscoring how important this principle is in shaping the world and the ecosystems around us.

The Natural Order and the Entropy of Ecosystems

Ecosystems, whether it's a dense forest or a vast ocean, are complex webs of life, where everything is interconnected. These natural systems are constantly balancing between order and chaos, and that balance is crucial for their health and resilience.

Consider a forest, for instance. It's a well-ordered system where everything has a role to play. Trees, plants, animals, and even the microorganisms in the soil work together, cycling nutrients and energy. This organization means low entropy; there's structure, purpose, and harmony within the system. Yet, disorder is never far off. In the natural world, entropy is always at work, but it's managed in a way that keeps ecosystems alive and thriving.

Natural processes like seasonal changes and evolutionary adaptations are key contributors to this balance. Take the changing of seasons, for example. As spring rolls in, plants burst into bloom, animals begin to reproduce, and ecosystems flourish. This is a time when order seems to prevail—everything works in sync to increase the complexity of life. But, as autumn and winter approach, the cycle reverses. Plants die back, animals hibernate, and the forest enters a phase of dormancy. It might seem like disorder has taken over, but in reality, this period of rest and decay is just nature's way of resetting and preparing for renewal. It's a balance—a rhythm of life and death, order and chaos.

Evolution, too, plays a vital role in this. Species evolve over time, adjusting to changing environments. It's a way for life to survive and adapt, keeping the natural order going even in the face of challenges. These adaptations, whether a bird develops stronger wings to migrate or a plant becomes more resilient to drought, are all part of maintaining that delicate balance within the ecosystem.

In stark contrast to the natural processes that maintain balance, human activities such as pollution, deforestation, and urban sprawl disrupt this delicate order and push ecosystems into a state of disorder that they are not equipped to handle. This is where the concept of entropy really comes to life, as our actions have introduced an unprecedented level of chaos into systems that once functioned with a degree of harmony.

Pollution is a prime example. The chemical products we use every day in the form of personal care items introduce pollutants into the environment. Even after treatment, trace amounts of these chemicals find their way into rivers, lakes, and oceans. This disrupts the oxygen levels in the water, suffocating aquatic life and creating a cascade of damage throughout the ecosystem. Here, human-induced entropy pushes natural systems beyond their ability to heal, leading to a decline in biodiversity and overall ecological health.

Moreover, the extraction and processing of raw materials, which fuel the production of these products, come with their own devastating consequences. Significant energy inputs are required, and often the process results in habitat destruction and soil degradation. These disruptions contribute to greater entropy by altering natural processes that are essential for maintaining ecological balance.

As the once-stable systems fall out of balance, the impact of increased entropy spreads, leading to environmental degradation on an ever-larger scale. To truly grasp the extent of how disrupting entropy affects our ecosystems, it's essential to step back and assess the massive, often unnoticed, impact. One of the most striking examples is the degradation of coral reefs, a case many of us have heard of but perhaps not fully understood in its gravity.

The Silent Collapse of Coral Reefs

Coral reefs, often referred to as the "rainforests of the sea," are among the most colorful and diverse ecosystems on the planet. Yet, they are under immense threat, primarily due to human-induced climate change, which has pushed the natural balance of entropy far beyond what these ecosystems can handle. Global warming, fueled by greenhouse gas emissions, has led to rising ocean temperatures, which trigger devastating coral bleaching events. When corals become stressed by higher temperatures, they expel the algae living within them—algae that provide essential nutrients to the corals. Without these algae, the corals lose their color, but more importantly, they lose their primary energy source, making survival increasingly difficult.

In addition to rising temperatures, ocean acidification, which is a direct result of increased carbon dioxide absorption, disrupts the very chemistry of seawater. Lower pH levels make it harder for corals to form their calcium carbonate skeletons, weakening the physical structures of reefs. This combination of warming and acidification accelerates the breakdown of coral ecosystems, increasing disorder and making it nearly impossible for them to recover naturally.

As these ecosystems weaken and collapse, so too do the livelihoods of those who depend on them. Coral reefs act as natural barriers, protecting coastlines from storms and erosion. Without them, communities become more vulnerable to the destructive forces of nature. The economic impact is also staggering, as many coastal areas thrive on tourism generated by the beauty and biodiversity of these reefs. When the reefs die, these communities lose a vital source of income.

This intricate balance, once disrupted, creates a feedback loop of disorder. The loss of coral reefs is a reminder of how increased entropy can unravel complex systems, throwing both nature and human society into a state of deeper imbalance.

The Consequences of Deforestation

Another significant example of human-induced disruption to natural entropy is deforestation, which has severe ecological and social consequences. Forests are vital in maintaining the delicate balance of ecosystems. They store carbon, regulate water cycles, and provide habitats for countless species. But when vast areas of forest are cleared for developing means of transportation, industrialization, or mining, this natural order is disrupted, pushing ecosystems toward disorder.

When trees are removed, especially through burning, the carbon stored in their trunks, branches, and leaves is released into the atmosphere as carbon dioxide, directly contributing to climate change. This increase in greenhouse gases accelerates global warming, creating a feedback loop of rising temperatures and shifting weather patterns. But the effects don't stop there.

The loss of forest cover affects the land and threatens the countless species that call these ecosystems home. When forests are cleared, habitats are destroyed, pushing species to the brink of extinction. This reduction in biodiversity weakens ecosystem resilience, making them less adaptable to environmental changes. In turn, this increases disorder within the ecosystem, making it harder for these natural systems to recover from disturbances.

Forests also play a critical role in protecting soil. Their roots hold the soil in place, preventing soil erosion, while the organic matter they shed enriches it, keeping it fertile and healthy. Without this cover, the soil is left exposed to the elements, vulnerable to erosion from wind and rain. Over time, this leads to a degradation of soil health, reducing its ability to support plant life. The loss of fertile soil affects not just local plant and animal life but also human communities that depend on the land for agriculture.

Many indigenous communities rely on forests for their livelihoods, traditions, and spiritual practices. The destruction of their lands impacts their economic well-being and erases a deep connection with the natural world, disrupting their way of life. Conflicts over land use often arise as the pressure to clear forests for agriculture or development grows, leaving these communities displaced and vulnerable.

In both cases, whether it's the degradation of coral reefs or the clearing of forests, human activities that increase entropy lead to destabilized ecosystems.

Restoring Balance

Once we fully understand our everyday choices, the harmful effects can be unsettling. It's no longer a question of whether we can change; it's a question of whether we're willing to do what it takes. This is about recognizing that the power to influence the world around us starts with the small, seemingly insignificant choices we make every day.

While we can't stop the natural laws of entropy from affecting the world, we have control over how much disorder we add. Every product we use and every choice we make either contributes to the chaos or helps restore balance. It's important to move beyond thinking solely about the direct effects on ourselves. When you step away from chemical-laden products, you begin to lessen the strain on ecosystems that are already under pressure. By choosing natural alternatives, you're taking care of both your health and the environment. The products we use on our bodies have an impact far beyond our immediate lives. Reducing synthetic compounds in our daily routines helps restore the balance in ecosystems, protecting them from further disruption.

This shift in mindset moves beyond changing what we buy—it's about rooted living. Each time you check an ingredient label or choose a product made with rooted living in mind, you are making a conscious decision to support a healthier world. It's about seeing the bigger picture, embracing awareness, and acting with purpose. It's a way of showing respect for our bodies, the planet, and future generations.

The beauty of making these conscious choices is how they start to resonate beyond your own life. As you make small, intentional shifts, others around you begin to notice. It sparks conversations, questions, and reflections. These changes can inspire your friends, family, and community to also reconsider their own habits, amplifying the impact far beyond what you initially imagined.

In the chapters ahead, I'll guide you through this transition step by step. Together, we'll uncover practical strategies to reduce the chaos we unknowingly introduce into our lives and the environment. Every chapter will take you through areas of your daily routine where chemical-laden products lurk and offer simple, natural alternatives that benefit both your health and the planet.

We'll start by looking at the basics: body cleansers like soaps and shampoos, and examine how switching to natural alternatives can not only clean and rejuvenate your skin but also reduce harmful impacts on water systems. From there, we'll move to facial care, exploring how the ingredients in everyday skincare products can affect you and entire ecosystems. Moving forward, we'll delve into the details of beauty routines, including lip balms, hand creams, and underarm care, and uncover how even small changes can dramatically reduce your environmental footprint. We'll address every part of your routine, from your hair to your legs, and find gentle, natural alternatives that are as effective as they are kind to the planet.

Finally, we'll bring it all together with a broader look at how our personal care, diets, and lifestyles can move toward more rooted and natural practices. The goal is to create a lifestyle that gives back to the environment, adopting a circular approach that mimics nature's cycles of renewal.

We now stand at the threshold of change. We've explored the hidden forces of entropy, how human choices disturb the natural order, and the impact that these disruptions have on our ecosystems, our health, and our future. With this understanding in hand, we are now ready to turn our focus towards the *how.*

I find Mother Teresa's words deeply fitting for this moment: "Yesterday is gone. Tomorrow has not yet come. We have only today. Let us begin." These words serve as a call to action. Today is where we start, where we decide to be more mindful of our bodies, our products, and our environment.

Section 2

Detox Your Routine, Heal the Planet

Chapter 6

Body Cleansing – Revisiting Our Routine

"Cleanliness is next to godliness."

It's one of those sayings we've all heard countless times. Think about this: you're visiting a serene temple or a peaceful sanctuary. The floors gleam, the air smells faintly of incense, and every corner reflects an almost sacred attention to care and detail. Now, think about how that environment feels- both physically pristine and spiritually uplifting. This connection between cleanliness and reverence is deeply integrated into how we've been taught to view care for our surroundings and, by extension, care for ourselves.

This deep-seated principle teaches us that treating our bodies with respect goes beyond superficial cleanliness; it's about honoring our physical selves in a way that mirrors the care we give to cherished, sacred places. However, as one looks at the abundance of brightly colored bottles of countless synthetic products, from cleansers and lotions to sprays and dyes, one can't help but question: Are we truly honoring our bodies in the way we have been taught? Have we perhaps strayed from the essence of this ancient wisdom?

It's a question that doesn't come naturally because we've been conditioned to believe that cleanliness is all about results: a spotless body, a fresh scent. But at what cost?

Those same bottles, filled with chemicals we barely recognize, are doing more than just washing away dirt. They're having a much bigger impact on our bodies and the environment. This is the conversation we need to have—not just about being clean but about being clean in a way that's aligned with nature, that respects the earth.

The Hidden Ingredients in Your Everyday Cleansers

Body washes and soaps are staples in our daily routines, but they often contain ingredients that many of us would struggle to pronounce, let alone understand. Ingredients like sodium lauryl sulfate (SLS), parabens, synthetic fragrances, triclosan, and artificial colorants are found in nearly every product we use for the sake of convenience and cleanliness. But what are these chemicals doing beyond just making us feel fresh?

Let's start with sodium lauryl sulfate (SLS), one of the most common ingredients in body washes and shampoos. It's the reason we get that rich, foamy lather that feels so satisfying. The foam gives the impression that we're getting squeaky clean, but SLS is a known skin irritant. If you've ever felt dryness or itchiness after a shower, especially if you have sensitive skin, this ingredient could be the culprit. And while we trust these products to be safe, studies suggest that SLS can be absorbed into the body, where it may disrupt our natural hormone balance.

Parabens are another common ingredient found in many body cleansers, often used for a practical reason: preservation. By preventing the growth of bacteria and mold, parabens extend the shelf life of products, keeping them fresh longer. While this might seem like a positive aspect on the surface, the health implications tell a different story. Parabens have been found to mimic estrogen, disrupting hormonal balance in the body, and are linked to an increased risk of breast cancer. What's troubling is the fact that studies have detected parabens in human tissues, showing that these chemicals can accumulate in our bodies over time. It's a sobering thought, especially considering how often we use these products.

Another key player in most body cleansers is synthetic fragrance. These fragrances make our soaps, shampoos, and body washes smell great, but at what cost? The term "fragrance" on a label can refer to hundreds of chemicals, many of which are hidden from consumers under that single word. One of the more concerning ingredients often found in synthetic fragrances is phthalates, chemicals known for disrupting the endocrine system, affecting reproductive health, and causing developmental issues. For people with sensitive skin, synthetic fragrances can also trigger allergic reactions or cause irritation, making these products more harmful than helpful.

Moving on to another worrisome chemical, triclosan, originally hailed for its antibacterial and antifungal properties, is still lurking in many personal care products despite its ban from antibacterial soaps by the FDA in 2016. Triclosan is known to interfere with thyroid function by disrupting hormones in the body, and there is also a significant issue with its link to antibiotic resistance. Despite the ban in some products, it still lingers in others, raising the question of whether we're unknowingly putting ourselves at risk. When triclosan interacts with chlorine in tap water, it can form chloroform, a chemical known to be a probable carcinogen.

Adding to the mix, artificial colorants are another common inclusion in many body cleansers. These synthetic dyes are used to make products visually appealing, but they are often derived from petroleum, which raises health and environmental concerns. While these colorants may not pose immediate harm in small concentrations, they can cause skin irritation or allergic reactions, especially for people with sensitive skin.

Beyond their effects on our skin, the environmental cost of producing and disposing of these synthetic dyes adds another layer to the issue. It's easy to see how the seemingly harmless products we use can have much deeper, more troubling effects when we dig a little further into their ingredients.

Environmental Effect of Chemical Cleansers

As we've seen, the ingredients in our body cleansers impact our bodies, but the environmental costs of producing these synthetic chemicals are just as alarming. Every time we reach for a bottle of body wash or shampoo, we are unknowingly supporting an industry that relies heavily on energy consumption, water pollution, soil pollution, and the depletion of natural resources.

The manufacturing process for these synthetic chemicals is energy-intensive, with many relying on non-renewable resources such as petroleum. Take, for example, sodium lauryl sulfate (SLS), that foaming agent we often associate with feeling clean. Its production requires complex chemical reactions, consuming vast amounts of energy and releasing carbon dioxide into the atmosphere. The carbon footprint of making these cleansers directly contributes to climate change, adding to the already overwhelming levels of greenhouse gases in our environment.

Water pollution is another serious issue tied to the production of these chemicals. Factories that manufacture synthetic ingredients for personal care products discharge wastewater filled with harmful substances into nearby rivers and lakes. This polluted water contains volatile organic compounds (VOCs), phthalates, and other toxic substances that accumulate in aquatic ecosystems. Despite modern wastewater treatment systems, many of these chemicals slip through the cracks and continue to harm the environment by mixing in the soil.

On top of water pollution and energy consumption, the depletion of natural resources adds another layer of environmental strain. Many of the ingredients in the body cleansers we use every day come from finite resources that are disappearing rapidly. For example, palm oil, which is often used to create sodium palmitate found in many soaps, comes at a great cost. The demand for palm oil has driven widespread deforestation in tropical regions, wiping out habitats and endangering countless species. The loss of these forests also means more carbon dioxide is released into the atmosphere, adding to the rising carbon emissions that accelerate climate change.

The mining of minerals like bauxite for aluminum-based compounds, which are found in some personal care products, also comes with devastating consequences. Mining practices often scar the land, disrupt local ecosystems, and degrade soil quality, leaving behind a trail of destruction that can take decades, if not longer, to heal.

The manufacturing process itself is a key contributor to environmental degradation, releasing toxic emissions and consuming immense amounts of energy. When chemicals like sodium lauryl sulfate (SLS) are produced, they require intense energy inputs through complex chemical reactions, often performed at high temperatures and pressures. The energy used in these processes typically comes from burning fossil fuels, which releases harmful carbon dioxide into the atmosphere and worsens the ongoing climate crisis.

While the manufacturing of body cleansers takes a significant toll on the environment, the problems don't stop once the products leave the factory. The environmental impact continues when we use these cleansers and wash them down the drain. Many of the chemicals, like sulfates and triclosan, find their way into our waterways, causing further damage to ecosystems.

When these chemicals are washed off our bodies and flow into wastewater treatment plants (WWTPs), the treatment facilities are often ill-equipped to fully remove them. As a result, they escape into rivers, lakes, and oceans, where they can cause serious harm to aquatic life. Sulfates, for example, are known to disrupt the natural balance of aquatic ecosystems, and the buildup of these chemicals in the water can have long-term consequences.

Triclosan is particularly problematic. It is highly persistent and can accumulate in waterways over time. Research shows that up to 96% of the triclosan from consumer products ends up in wastewater treatment plants. Although some of it is filtered out, a significant amount remains in the water. Worse, triclosan can undergo chemical reactions during the treatment process, forming even more dangerous compounds like dioxins. These toxic byproducts are nearly impossible to break down and can poison aquatic environments, posing a serious risk to marine life and potentially entering the food chain.

The broader environmental concerns stretch beyond water. Triclosan and other chemicals convert into compounds like dioxins, known for their persistence and toxicity. These compounds can contaminate soil and air, affecting plant life and wildlife. They can even enter our food system through plants irrigated with polluted water, bringing these chemicals right back to our dinner tables. The interconnectedness between the products we use, the environment, and our own well-being becomes alarmingly clear.

Embracing Natural Alternatives

The impact of chemical cleansers on both our bodies and the environment leaves us searching for alternatives that align with the idea of rooted living—living in harmony with nature, making choices that nurture rather than harm. This is where natural cleansers come in. Made from plant-based ingredients like food grains, flowers, fruits, oils, herbal extracts, and natural fats, these alternatives offer a path forward that is kinder to both the planet and our bodies in and out.

One of the most important aspects of these natural products is their ability to break down easily in the environment. Unlike the synthetic chemicals found in conventional body cleansers, natural ingredients like rice and gram powder, oil, and aloe vera gel decompose into harmless substances when washed down the drain. This biodegradability means that, instead of leaving behind toxic residues, these cleansers simply return to the earth without polluting our water systems.

What does this mean for our rivers, lakes, and oceans? It means a cleaner, healthier environment for aquatic life. Natural cleansers avoid harmful additives such as sulfates, parabens, and synthetic fragrances—chemicals that often disrupt the balance of aquatic ecosystems. Instead, they use natural surfactants, derived from plants or animal fats, which don't harm the protective mucus layers of fish or disturb the water quality.

In addition to the benefits for our waterways, the production of natural cleansing products brings its own set of environmental advantages. Compared to synthetic chemicals, the manufacturing processes for natural ingredients are simpler and less energy-consuming. Extracting oils from plants or creating herbal formulations requires fewer steps and less energy, which means fewer greenhouse gases are emitted. This is a stark contrast to the energy-intensive production of synthetic chemicals, which often relies on fossil fuels and complex processes. By choosing natural cleansers, you're also making a direct impact on reducing the carbon footprint of your daily routine.

Beyond the environmental benefits, natural cleansers offer something uniquely valuable for your skin. Free from the harsh chemicals that can irritate and disrupt, they are enriched with phytonutrients, vitamins, and antioxidants—gifts directly from nature. These ingredients provide nourishment and support the skin's health, transforming the act of cleaning into an act of caring. It's a shift in mindset, from stripping away to nurturing what's already there.

This natural approach to cleansing is especially considerate of the differences in our skin types. For instance, a blend of rice powder and aloe vera gel offers a soothing, hydrating cleanse for those with dry or sensitive skin, utilizing the gentle exfoliation of rice powder combined with the moisturizing properties of aloe vera. On the other hand, a mix of besan and rice powder could be ideal for those needing deeper exfoliation, helping to remove dead skin cells and brighten the complexion without over-drying.

Whether you're dealing with oily skin that benefits from the oil-absorbing properties of Multani mitti and the soothing effects of chandan powder, or combination skin that requires the balancing act of besan mixed with nourishing rose powder, natural cleansers can be tailored to meet these needs effectively. Each ingredient is selected both for its functional benefits and its alignment with a lifestyle that respects both body and planet.

These examples show how natural products work so well with our unique skin, giving you a more personal experience and fitting perfectly with a rooted lifestyle.

When I use natural cleansers, I'll admit that it's a bit time consuming. I have spent a lot of time with many products, testing different combinations, and figuring out what worked best for my skin. To make this process easier for you, I've compiled a few simple, natural alternatives that are easy to incorporate into your body cleansing routine. These options can leave you feeling fresher and happier— way better than a spa experience.

Shower with Rice Powder Body Scrubber

Rice powder is a gentle yet effective exfoliant, packed with antioxidants and nutrients that nourish the skin while removing dead cells and impurities. It leaves your skin feeling smooth and refreshed. You can make a rice powder body scrub at home by mixing rice flour with either honey, oil, or lemon juice. Honey adds moisture, and the lemon provides a natural brightening effect, thanks to its vitamin C. Simply apply in gentle, circular motions and rinse off, leaving your skin feeling soft and renewed. If you add any oil of your choice to this mix, you don't need to moisturize your skin post-shower.

Shower with Rice and Masoor Powder Blend

A combination of rice flour and masoor dal powder works wonders as a natural cleanser. Masoor dal is full of vitamins and minerals that cleanse and exfoliate while also helping to brighten the skin. To create this at home, grind equal parts of rice and masoor dal into a fine powder, mix it with water or rose water to make a smooth paste, add some oil, and the mix is ready. This blend helps in reducing tan, evening out skin tone, and giving your skin a natural glow.

Shower with Masoor Dal Paste

Masoor dal paste is another fantastic option for deep cleansing and exfoliation. Rich in antioxidants, this paste helps combat skin damage and nourish your skin. To make it, soak masoor dal overnight, grind it into a smooth paste the next morning, and add oil. This can be applied to your skin to gently scrub away dirt and impurities, leaving it feeling fresh and rejuvenated. Over time, you might also notice a brighter complexion and fewer signs of aging, as this natural remedy helps minimize wrinkles and promotes healthy, glowing skin.

Shower with Besan Paste

Besan, or gram flour, has been a trusted natural cleanser for generations. It's excellent for balancing pH levels and removing excess oil while exfoliating dead skin cells. To make this simple yet effective paste, mix besan with water or yogurt until smooth. You can use this all over your face and body for a thorough, refreshing cleanse that leaves your skin feeling clean and soft.

Shower with Besan and Rice Powder Mix

For an even deeper exfoliation, try combining besan with rice powder. This blend works wonders for removing dead skin cells and brightening your complexion. Mix equal parts of besan and rice powder with water to create a scrub. Gently massage it into your skin and rinse off to reveal a smoother, more radiant appearance.

Shower with Besan and Chandan Powder

The combination of besan (gram flour) and chandan (sandalwood powder) brings together the deep-cleansing properties of besan with the calming, anti-inflammatory effects of chandan. This blend is especially effective for reducing acne, scars, and redness, making it a great option for irritated or blemish-prone skin. Mix these two with rose water to create a paste, apply it as a mask, and feel the soothing relief as your skin absorbs the natural goodness.

Shower with Besan and Rose Powder

If you're looking for something that's effective and leaves a delicate, refreshing fragrance, besan with rose powder is a wonderful choice. Rose powder has anti-inflammatory properties that soothe irritation while hydrating your skin. Mixing besan with rose powder and a little milk creates a gentle cleanser that leaves your skin soft and smelling lovely, while the rose powder works to calm and refresh your skin.

Shower with Multani Mitti Powder

Multani mitti, or fuller's earth, is a well-known natural clay that has been used for ages to tackle oily skin. It's fantastic for absorbing excess oil, clearing up acne, and brightening the skin. All you need is to mix multani mitti with water or rose water to make a smooth paste, which acts as an excellent mask for clearing impurities and evening out your skin tone.

Shower with Multani Mitti and Chandan Powder

Pairing multani mitti with chandan powder gives you a deeper, more enriching cleanse. This combination helps reduce pigmentation while soothing irritated skin. Mix these two powders with water to create a paste, and use it as a mask to reveal clear, glowing skin.

Shower with Aloe Vera Gel and Rice Powder

Finally, for those with dry or sensitive skin, aloe vera gel combined with rice powder is an ideal solution. Aloe vera is renowned for its soothing and hydrating properties, making it a perfect partner for rice powder's gentle exfoliation. This blend provides a moisturizing yet exfoliating experience, leaving your skin feeling soft and nourished. Simply mix the aloe vera gel and rice powder into a paste and take a shower with this mixture.

What I do is create the shower mixtures in different bottles for a month or two at a time and customize them by adding oil, saffron, orange peel powder, rose petal powder, or lemon juice, depending on the season, mood, and time for the shower.

Your Path to Natural Cleansing

After exploring these natural alternatives, you might be feeling inspired to make the switch and start your own journey toward more sustainable and skin-friendly cleansers. The good news is that transitioning to these natural cleansers is simple as they are mostly from your kitchen.

The first step in this process is understanding what's currently in the products you use. Take a moment to check the ingredient list on your body cleansers, soaps, and shampoos. You'll likely find a number of chemicals like sulfates, parabens, and synthetic fragrances that we've discussed. Once you've decided to cut the chemicals from your cleansing routine, it's time to choose natural alternatives that suit your skin type. If you have sensitive skin, you may want to start with gentler options like rice powder scrubs or besan pastes, which cleanse and exfoliate without irritating your skin. Balance by adding oil depending on the nature of your skin based on oil secretion.

A good way to begin this transition is to replace one product at a time. This gradual approach gives your skin a chance to adjust to new ingredients. Start with something you use daily, like your body wash or soap. With this first step, I am sure you will start feeling more connected to your body and the plant.

Chapter 7

Facial Care – Protecting Our Visage

When you look in the mirror, what do you see? More than just features, you see the very essence of who you are. Your face is a powerful canvas that tells your story to the world. It reflects joy, sorrow, love, and even the journey you've walked. Every laugh line and every freckle carries a piece of your life, a memory that speaks to others without words. And that's why how we care for our face goes far beyond the surface.

Facial care is about treating this remarkable part of ourselves with the respect and attention it deserves. Just as we wouldn't treat a sacred space casually, our face deserves mindful, thoughtful care that nurtures its health and vitality. This means choosing products that don't just sit on the skin or promise quick fixes but that truly nourish and support our skin's natural needs.

The skin on our faces is more sensitive and delicate. It interacts daily with the world around us, weathering the elements, showing our emotions, and holding our expressions. When we reach for a product, it's a choice: do we choose something that respects and cares for our face or something that might harm it?

Beginning this journey of caring for our faces with the respect they deserve, it's worth acknowledging how the beauty industry has shaped our routines and, often, our perceptions. Our faces have become a primary focus for cosmetic brands, which have skillfully tapped into our desire to care for and enhance this vital part of ourselves. But the industry's influence goes beyond offering simple solutions; it strategically shapes our habits, playing on beauty ideals to promote products we're told are essential for flawless, youthful skin.

This focus is a deliberate effort to capitalize on cultural standards of beauty. We see countless ads and social media posts presenting smooth, glowing skin as the ultimate goal, creating a narrative that our worth is somehow tied to how closely we fit these ideals. This messaging normalizes complex, multi-step routines with cleansers, serums, toners, and more. In 2022, the beauty industry raked in a staggering $430 billion worldwide, with skincare capturing a big chunk of that. This really shows just how deeply beauty ideals are woven into our everyday lives.

Yet, as we layer on these products, we rarely consider the impact of the ingredients within them. Many contain chemicals designed to deliver quick results, but their long-term effects on our skin and the world around us are less reassuring. Our skin absorbs much of what we apply, allowing chemicals to enter our bodies and potentially disrupt our natural balance.

The Chemical Facade in Facial Care

It's eye-opening to realize what goes into the facial products we trust daily as we peel back the layers of the beauty industry's influence. Let's look closely at some of the most common chemical ingredients that have found their way into our routines, embedded in our creams, serums, and cleansers. These aren't just random scientific names you find on ingredient labels; each one serves a specific purpose—whether it's improving texture, keeping products fresh, or locking in scents. However, these seemingly harmless chemicals also raise some important concerns that we need to pay attention to.

Phthalates, for instance, are often present in fragrances. They work as fixatives, helping scents last longer, but phthalates are known to be readily absorbed into the skin, building up over time. Research has shown that they can interfere with our hormonal systems, potentially leading to imbalances that disrupt normal bodily functions. Over time, these disruptions raise questions about long-term health impacts, particularly regarding endocrine health.

Then we have parabens, which you might recognize, as they've become infamous in recent years. Added to facial care products to prevent bacterial growth, parabens keep items from spoiling. But this preservative effect may come at a cost. Studies have pointed out that parabens can accumulate in our bodies, disrupting cellular functions and affecting the skin's health. For example, methylparaben, a common paraben variant, has been found to alter skin cells and potentially contribute to premature aging by diminishing skin cell renewal.

Now, let's turn to synthetic fragrances, which are often marketed to elevate the skincare experience. Beneath their appealing scents, however, lies a mixture of complex chemicals that can provoke various health concerns. These fragrances are typically composed of compounds known to cause skin allergies, like benzene derivatives and formaldehyde-releasing agents, both of which can increase skin sensitivity. For those prone to dermatitis or other allergic reactions, the use of products with synthetic fragrances may lead to flare-ups and persistent irritation.

Another frequent ingredient, polyethylene glycols (PEGs), serves as an emulsifier, creating a smooth consistency in many facial care products. However, PEGs can strip the skin of its natural oils, leaving it vulnerable to dryness and compromised. When the skin barrier weakens, it loses some of its defenses against environmental factors, making it more susceptible to irritation and damage over time.

Alcohols, which are often present in facial cleansers and toners, add a quick-drying quality that can feel refreshing but, in reality, can be too harsh on the skin. Alcohols like ethanol tend to strip away natural oils, leading to a drying effect that can compound over repeated use. This is especially challenging for those with naturally dry or sensitive skin, as it can accelerate dehydration and cause discomfort.

Lastly, silicones are frequently included in facial care products to provide that silky, smooth texture we're accustomed to. While they do create a barrier that locks in moisture, this layer can also trap dirt and sebum, leading to clogged pores and potentially triggering breakouts. For many, the prolonged use of silicone-heavy products can weigh on the skin, leading to a cycle of clogged pores and blemishes.

The daily exposure to these substances, layer upon layer, can result in a range of skin issues over time. This raises an important question for us as consumers: How can we balance the need for effective skincare with an understanding of the ingredients we're using? Knowing what goes into our products helps us make mindful choices that support both immediate skin health and long-term well-being.

The Impact Beyond the Bathroom Sink

Moving on from the personal impacts on our skin to the broader environmental picture, it's essential to understand the toll these chemicals take on our planet. From the initial production of ingredients like silicones, phthalates, and parabens to the final disposal of these products, the environmental footprint is massive. The manufacturing processes for these chemicals are energy-heavy and leave a considerable carbon footprint, intensifying climate change. Take silicones, for instance. Creating silicones requires extracting silicon from silica, a process involving high-temperature reduction using coal or charcoal. This consumes huge amounts of energy and releases significant levels of carbon dioxide into the atmosphere.

Adding to this are the layers of transportation and distribution that these products undergo before they land on store shelves. The beauty industry's supply chain is extensive, involving raw material extraction, chemical processing, and global product distribution. Each stage releases emissions, often referred to as Scope 3 emissions, which make up a substantial portion of the beauty industry's overall carbon footprint. These emissions are complex to track and control, yet their impact on climate is substantial.

We also need to address the impact of disposing of them. Imagine the lifecycle of your favorite face wash or sunscreen—it doesn't end when the product washes down the drain. Ingredients like silicones and synthetic compounds linger in our environment because they aren't biodegradable. They often find their way into rivers, lakes, and oceans, where they can stick around for years, disrupting marine life.

Wastewater treatment facilities struggle to remove these chemicals, so they enter our natural water systems and even pose dangers as endocrine disruptors to wildlife. Sunscreens are a prime example of good intentions with unintended consequences. Ingredients designed to protect us from the sun, such as oxybenzone and octinoxate, wash off during a swim or shower and persist in waterways. Their stability and fat-soluble nature make them particularly problematic, especially in coastal regions bustling with tourists. Here, sunscreen use accumulates in the water, dramatically affecting local ecosystems.

The effects of ingredients like oxybenzone and octinoxate in sunscreens become even more alarming when we consider their role as endocrine disruptors. hey function as endocrine disruptors, meaning they interfere with the delicate hormonal balance of marine life. This effect is particularly destructive in coral reefs, where these chemicals disrupt the vital partnership between corals and the algae living within them. This symbiotic relationship is essential to coral survival; when disrupted, it leads to coral bleaching. In such events, corals lose their vibrant colors and, more critically, their strength, leaving them vulnerable to disease and, ultimately, death.

The reach of these chemicals doesn't stop with coral. Oxybenzone and octinoxate can bioaccumulate—meaning they build up within the bodies of marine species like fish and mollusks. This accumulation affects these creatures' reproductive health and growth, posing a broader threat to the biodiversity of the entire marine ecosystem. Each species affected can have a cascading impact on the food web, affecting ecosystem stability on multiple levels.

In response, some places, including Hawaii and Key West, have taken a strong stance, banning the sale of sunscreens containing these harmful UV filters. These measures serve as a wake-up call, emphasizing the need for safer, more natural alternatives in the products we use.

Embracing Purity with Natural Facial Care

Reflecting on the impact of chemical-laden facial products on both our skin and the environment, we see that a shift toward natural facial care is necessary and deeply empowering. This shift is rooted in the idea of "rooted living," which aligns with both our bodies' natural rhythms and the environment around us. By choosing ingredients that work with our skin rather than against it, we give our faces the kind of care that respects their natural processes.

Natural ingredients bring a host of benefits. Oils, plant extracts, and essential nutrients offer gentle support to the skin's natural barrier, preserving moisture while reducing the likelihood of irritation and dryness. Ingredients like jojoba oil, rosehip oil, and shea butter nourish deeply without disrupting the delicate balance of our skin. These elements are rich in vitamins, antioxidants, and fatty acids that encourage repair and promote a healthy, resilient complexion.

One of the wonderful things about using natural ingredients is their versatility. They can be easily adapted to meet the unique needs of different skin types. For example, aloe vera gel provides lightweight hydration, making it ideal for those with oily or acne-prone skin. Meanwhile, those with sensitive or dry skin may find that richer oils, like shea butter or almond oil, provide a calming, deep moisture that softens and soothes.

Switching to natural facial care also helps reduce the risks associated with long-term exposure to synthetic chemicals. Conventional skincare products often contain preservatives, synthetic fragrances, and additives that can disturb the skin's natural balance, sometimes causing irritation or even allergic reactions over time. By moving toward natural ingredients, we can avoid many of these risks while still keeping our skin healthy and vibrant.

Additionally, natural facial care products often come with a smaller environmental footprint, as they are typically biodegradable and sourced from renewable resources. Unlike synthetic chemicals that can linger in ecosystems, natural ingredients break down more easily, reducing the environmental strain that chemical-laden products can cause.

To start exploring natural options that truly care for both us and our environment, let's take a look at a few standout ingredients for the first process of facial care, i.e., cleaning. The good thing about all the options below is that you can use them as a cleanser and as a face pack too.

Aloe Vera Gel is known for its calming and hydrating properties, making it an excellent choice across all skin types, especially for those with sensitive or acne-prone skin. Lightweight and non-greasy, it hydrates without clogging pores, bringing soothing moisture that's perfect for daily use. Packed with vitamins A, C, and E, aloe vera works to neutralize free radicals, aiding in skin repair and boosting collagen production, which helps improve elasticity and smooths out fine lines. Thanks to its anti-inflammatory benefits, aloe vera can calm irritated skin and reduce redness, making it a go-to for soothing sunburns or inflamed acne. To enjoy its benefits, simply massage the gel onto clean skin and leave it on for 10-15 minutes before rinsing. For those with oily skin, aloe vera acts as a gentle astringent, keeping excess oil in check and reducing breakouts. You can also mix it with honey for an antibacterial boost or turmeric for a brightening effect.

Raw Milk offers a wealth of skin-loving vitamins and minerals, bringing gentle exfoliation and hydration. Rich in lactic acid, raw milk delicately removes dead skin cells, leaving the skin fresh and radiant. Raw milk is one of the best ways to cleanse your face. Vitamins A, D, and E, along with essential fatty acids, provide much-needed nourishment, making raw milk ideal for dry or sensitive skin. Its lactic acid content also contributes to mild exfoliation, helping to smooth the skin's texture and reveal a brighter complexion. Applying raw milk directly to the face as a gentle cleanser or mixing it into masks can improve hydration and provide a noticeable glow, revealing fresh, soft skin beneath.

Curd, or yogurt, is packed with probiotics and lactic acid, making it a versatile addition to any facial care routine. The probiotics in curd support the skin's natural microbiome, ensuring a balanced and healthy complexion. The lactic acid acts as a mild exfoliant, gently sloughing off dead skin cells to reveal a smoother, more radiant surface. Suitable for both oily and dry skin types, curd helps balance moisture while reducing acne and blemishes, thanks to its anti-inflammatory properties. Applying it is simple—use it as a face mask, leaving it on for 15-20 minutes before rinsing. Mixing curd with honey adds extra hydration, while a touch of turmeric boosts its antibacterial qualities, creating a nourishing mask that leaves your skin calm and refreshed.

Rice Paste is another ingredient known for its ability to absorb excess oil and gently exfoliate the skin. Rich in starch, rice paste is particularly beneficial for oily or combination skin, as it helps control sebum while soothing any redness or irritation. To incorporate it, blend rice flour with water or rose water to form a smooth paste, applying it to the skin and letting it dry before rinsing. The result is a tightened, brighter complexion that feels clean and renewed. You can also mix it with milk or aloe vera to boost hydration and enhance its calming effects.

Gram Flour (Besan) is a traditional skincare staple, known for its deep cleansing and exfoliating properties. Gram flour is rich in zinc, helping to manage oiliness and reduce acne by absorbing excess oil and unclogging pores. Ideal for oily and combination skin, it's an effective way to cleanse and brighten naturally. To use, mix besan with yogurt or rose water into a paste, applying it as a face mask and allowing it to dry before gently scrubbing off with water. This purifies and smoothens skin texture by removing dead cells and impurities. Adding turmeric elevates its antibacterial properties, making it especially effective against breakouts.

Masoor Dal Paste stands out as an exceptional natural exfoliant and cleanser, especially beneficial for dry or maturing skin. Rich in essential nutrients, it enhances the skin's elasticity and diminishes the appearance of fine lines. To prepare this nourishing paste, soak masoor dal overnight and grind it into a fine mixture. Apply it as a mask or a scrub to cleanse and refresh your complexion. For an extra boost of hydration, you can enrich the paste with milk or honey, enhancing its moisturizing benefits.

Urad Dal Paste is another excellent choice, particularly for those with dry or sensitive skin. Its gentle exfoliating properties remove dead skin cells without causing irritation, thanks to its fine texture and nourishing components. Urad dal, abundant in proteins and vitamins, fortifies the skin's barrier, enhancing its overall health and resilience. To integrate urad dal into your skincare ritual, soak the dal overnight and blend it into a smooth paste. For a soothing touch, mix it with yogurt or rose water before applying it to your face as a calming mask or scrub.

Potato Juice offers a natural solution for brightening the complexion and reducing dark spots. Known for its mild bleaching effects, potato juice is rich in vitamins C and B6, which hydrate and soothe the skin while minimizing inflammation. This makes it a superb option for those looking to even out their skin tone, particularly if they have hyperpigmentation. To harness the benefits of potato juice, grate a potato and squeeze out the juice. Apply it directly to affected areas or enhance its efficacy with a splash of lemon juice for additional brightening. Leave it on the skin for about 15-20 minutes before rinsing off to reveal a more luminous complexion.

Orange Peel Powder is a fantastic addition, especially for those with oily or dull skin. Packed with vitamin C, this powder works as a natural exfoliant, effectively brightening the skin by sloughing away dead cells. Its antioxidants actively combat free radicals, enhancing your skin's natural glow. To create a refreshing mask, blend orange peel powder with yogurt or honey, applying the mixture to your face and letting it dry before rinsing off. This simple step can leave your skin looking revitalized and feeling refreshed, with a brightness that only nature can provide.

Fuller's Earth (Multani Mitti), a clay treasured for its exceptional oil-absorbing properties, is perfect for oily or acne-prone skin. This natural clay draws out impurities from pores, cleansing deeply while leaving your skin cool and refreshed. Multani Mitti's calming effects are especially soothing for inflamed skin. To incorporate it into your facial care, mix Fuller's Earth with water or rose water to create a smooth paste, applying it as a mask and allowing it to dry before rinsing with lukewarm water. For an even more enriching experience, try blending it with sandalwood powder or aloe vera gel to amplify its cleansing and soothing effects.

Making the Switch

Transitioning from chemical-based facial care to natural products is a journey that brings rewards for both your skin and the environment. To make this transition as smooth and enjoyable as possible, here are some practical tips to guide you through each step.

Understanding Your Skin's Needs

The first step in choosing natural alternatives is to understand your skin's unique qualities. Take a closer look at your skin type—whether it tends to be oily, dry, a combination of both, or sensitive. Think about specific needs too, like dealing with breakouts, addressing uneven tone, or simply aiming for a bit more glow. Having a clear picture of your skin's preferences will help you choose the natural ingredients that can best address these needs.

Ease into Natural Products Gradually

Switching everything at once can overwhelm your skin, so take it slow with a gradual replacement approach. Start by swapping out the products that have the most contact with your skin, like cleansers and moisturizers, and introduce them one at a time over a few weeks. This way, your skin can adapt without feeling 'shocked' by the new ingredients. You'll also be able to tell which products work best for you, one at a time.

Anticipate a Detox Phase

As your skin adjusts to natural ingredients, it might go through a short detox phase. This is completely normal—think of it as your skin releasing old buildup from chemical products. During this time, you might notice breakouts or slight oiliness, but it's usually temporary. Keeping this in mind can help you stick with the transition without frustration, knowing it's part of the process toward healthier skin.

Educating Yourself on Natural Ingredients

As with any worthwhile journey, knowledge is key. Learning about various natural ingredients will help you understand which options suit your unique skincare needs. Take some time to explore the benefits of ingredients like aloe vera, honey, and oils, and experiment with mixing them with the options listed above to learn what's best for you in terms of ease and your face. These ingredients have a range of properties, from soothing and hydrating to balancing and revitalizing.

Making a Long-Term Commitment

Embracing a natural skincare routine is truly a long-term choice. While you may not see instant results, the gentle, consistent effects of natural ingredients are worth the wait. Natural products don't aim to deliver quick fixes; rather, they nurture the skin over time, leading to lasting benefits. Patience and consistency will be your allies, and as you stay committed, you'll notice healthier skin that reflects your dedication to this journey.

Each thoughtful choice in your natural skincare routine contributes to your well-being and to a broader commitment to environmental balance.

Chapter 8

Face Focus – Eyes to Lips

In today's world, facial skincare has taken on a life of its own, urging us to think about our faces in pieces rather than as a single, cohesive whole. Just take a look at any skincare aisle, and you'll see what I mean: there are creams dedicated just for the under-eye area, gels for the eyebrows and toners for the nose. It's a collection of products for every part of our face, each with a unique promise to "solve" the specific needs of that area.

This shift didn't come out of nowhere. It's driven by consumer demand, and the relentless marketing that convinces us each part of our face has its own set of problems—ones that, apparently, need their own distinct chemical solutions. So, these days, we end up piling on a ton of products every day, way past the old simple cleanse-and-moisturize routine that used to be the go-to.

Social media and influencer culture have taken this skincare trend to new heights. On platforms like Instagram and TikTok, beauty influencers showcase their intricate routines, packed with numerous steps and specialized products targeting different areas of the face. They make it all seem so effortless and essential, convincing many of us that we need a product for every tiny "flaw" we spot in the mirror.

But there's a hidden side to this beauty routine boom. Many people dive into these multi-step routines without fully realizing the impact of layering so many different chemicals on their skin. So, before adding yet another product to the shelf, it's worth considering a more rooted approach, one that treats our face as a whole rather than a collection of individual problems.

The Hidden Ingredients in Eye Care Products

To really grasp how these products affect us and the environment, we need to dig deeper and uncover the true costs they impose on our health and the planet. Let's begin by looking at what we put around our eyes, and then we can explore other common areas of facial care, like our lips and nose.

Eye products like eyebrow pencils, gels, mascaras, eyeshadows, and eyeliners are formulated with a range of synthetic waxes, microplastics, and petroleum-based polymers. These substances help give our makeup that desirable smooth application, long wear, and defined look. But there's more lurking beneath the surface of these seemingly harmless beauty enhancers.

Take eyebrow pencils and gels, for example. These products are carefully blended with waxes, oils, and pigments to give a sleek and consistent application. However, the waxes used in many of these formulas are often synthetic, such as polyethylene or silicone-based waxes, which come from petroleum. This connects these products to the extraction of non-renewable fossil fuels, and it also means that the waste from these ingredients contributes to pollution when they are washed off or thrown away.

Following eyebrow pencils and gels, mascaras and eyelid makeup like eyeshadows and eyeliners are equally dependent on synthetic polymers and microplastics to achieve popular effects like enhanced volume, shimmer, and longer-lasting wear. These products often contain glittery or glossy particles that contribute significantly to plastic pollution, especially when washed down the drain.

The glitter in eyeshadows and eyeliners, for example, is usually crafted from materials like polyethylene terephthalate (PET) or polyvinyl chloride (PVC)—forms of plastic that are incredibly small, often less than 5 millimeters, making them very difficult to filter out during wastewater treatment. These microplastics ultimately make their way into rivers, lakes, and oceans, where they become a lasting environmental hazard.

Once in aquatic ecosystems, these microplastics pose serious risks to marine life. Fish, plankton, and other marine organisms often mistake these tiny particles for food, unknowingly ingesting them. Over time, microplastics accumulate within their digestive systems, leading to several health issues. For instance, the particles can block their digestive tracts, preventing them from eating enough actual food, which can lead to malnutrition. Additionally, studies reveal that microplastics can alter natural feeding behaviors, reduce reproductive rates, and even damage internal organs in marine species. As these microplastics move up the food chain—from plankton to small fish to larger predators—the concentration of these toxins intensifies, a process known as biomagnification. This buildup threatens marine biodiversity and raises health risks for us, too, as these contaminated particles ultimately make their way to our tables through seafood.

The spread of microplastics is so pervasive that no part of the ocean, not even the most remote corners, is untouched by this pollution. Their reach reveals a troubling truth about our cosmetic choices and the long-lasting impact they have on ecosystems far beyond our immediate surroundings.

Apart from microplastics, many cosmetic products contain petroleum-based ingredients, such as mineral oils or petrolatum, which create smooth textures and long-lasting effects in makeup formulas. However, the environmental cost of extracting and refining petroleum is high. The petroleum industry significantly contributes to greenhouse gas emissions and pollution, underscoring the ecological impact that goes into creating even a single tube of mascara or jar of cream. Furthermore, these ingredients can clog pores and sometimes cause skin irritation or allergic reactions.

As we examine the ingredients in our eye care routines, another problematic component surfaces: mica. Known for its signature shimmer, mica lends a luminous quality to countless products, especially under-eye cosmetics, eyeshadows, and highlighters. But the shine we seek in these products has a hidden cost, especially for the ecosystems and communities where mica is mined.

The extraction of mica, particularly in countries like India, Madagascar, and Brazil, comes at an immense environmental cost. Mined primarily through open-pit methods, mica extraction involves stripping away large areas of vegetation and topsoil, a process that results in severe deforestation and long-term environmental degradation. In places like Jharkhand in India, forests have been cleared to make room for expansive mica mining operations, disrupting entire ecosystems. Wildlife, including elephants, wild boars, and rare birds, are forced to leave or face extinction due to the loss of their natural habitats. The impact of these losses damages the biodiversity essential to these regions, pushing species to the brink as their homes are destroyed.

Beyond deforestation, the environmental toll of mica mining seeps into the land and local communities. When vegetation is stripped away, the soil loses its stability, making it vulnerable to erosion and landslides. This disrupts the land's natural balance and compromises its fertility, affecting local communities that rely on the land for agriculture and sustenance. The open-pit mining also destabilizes underground layers, leading to the formation of sinkholes, which pose a serious threat to the lives of nearby residents and wildlife alike.

Let's look at another layer—the pigments and synthetic compounds in eyebrow pencils, eyeshadows, and under-eye products. While pigments like iron oxides and titanium dioxide are often used for color, they can be accompanied by harmful additives such as coal tar derivatives or heavy metals. Over time, these substances can accumulate in the human body, potentially affecting internal organs and overall health. And once they enter the environment through wastewater, titanium dioxide, in particular, becomes a disruptor. Reflecting sunlight underwater, this compound interferes with photosynthesis for aquatic plants and coral reefs, a process essential for underwater life and oxygen generation.

Under-eye products like creams and serums also introduce complex chemicals into our ecosystems. Ingredients such as caffeine, retinol derivatives, and silicone compounds are added for their ability to target concerns like puffiness, wrinkles, and dark circles. However, the long-term impact of these ingredients on our environment often goes unnoticed. Caffeine, for example, is widely used for its ability to constrict blood vessels and reduce puffiness around the eyes. But once washed off, caffeine often persists in wastewater, flowing into rivers and lakes where it can disturb aquatic ecosystems. Even in small concentrations, caffeine acts as a stimulant, affecting hormonal cycles in fish and amphibians, which can alter their reproductive behaviors and disrupt delicate population balances. For instance, fish that typically control algae populations may see reproductive shifts, and amphibians—critical both as predators and prey in their ecosystems—may experience changes up the food chain.

These choices, made in the name of self-care, therefore have larger consequences. While they promise beauty benefits, they simultaneously contribute to an unseen but powerful wave of disruption in ecosystems, affecting species that keep the environment in balance.

Lip Care Products: The Hidden Impact Behind the Gloss

Having considered the effects of eye makeup on both our health and the environment, let's turn to another everyday beauty staple—lip care products. Lipsticks and lip glosses, loved for their aesthetic appeal, hold a hidden layer of risks that goes far beyond just looking good. The chemicals used in these products, including synthetic dyes, petroleum-based ingredients, parabens, and fragrances, can have a considerable impact on both our bodies and the world around us.

The delicate skin on our lips is especially vulnerable to chemicals due to its unique makeup. Without the protection of sweat glands or hair follicles, lips are more permeable, meaning they easily absorb whatever is applied to them. This permeability allows chemicals from lip products to enter the body more readily, which can lead to various skin issues over time. Prolonged use of lip products containing synthetic dyes or fragrances, for example, can result in dryness, cracking, and even allergic reactions. A condition known as cheilitis—marked by inflammation and irritation of the lips—often stems from repeated exposure to these substances. Studies indicate that common side effects include hyperpigmentation, a persistent burning sensation, and, for some users, even the formation of pustules. These are issues that affect comfort, appearance, and overall skin health.

There's a deeper layer when we examine the environmental impact of their ingredients. One of the most troubling components in lipsticks is the use of synthetic pigments, particularly azo dyes. These synthetic colorants, responsible for the bold reds, pinks, and oranges so popular in cosmetics, bring with them more than just vibrant color. While azo dyes are chosen for their brightness and staying power, their environmental toll is severe. When they wash off or are discarded, they find their way into our water systems, where they degrade into compounds called aromatic amines. Some of these breakdown products are recognized as carcinogens, adding to the pollution burden on natural habitats.

Azo dyes are notoriously resistant to breaking down, meaning they persist in aquatic environments for extended periods. Wastewater treatment plants often struggle to remove them completely, leaving remnants that continue to circulate through water systems. Once in lakes, rivers, or oceans, these dyes disrupt biological cycles, particularly by blocking light penetration in water bodies. This reduction in light limits photosynthesis in aquatic plants and algae, which play a crucial role in producing oxygen for aquatic ecosystems. As photosynthesis decreases, oxygen levels drop, creating hypoxic conditions that can severely impact fish populations and other aquatic life.

Studies also reveal that azo dyes are acutely toxic to many aquatic species, causing growth reduction, metabolic strain, and even damage to neurosensory systems in fish and amphibians. These species are integral to their ecosystems—many control insect populations or serve as prey for larger animals. When their populations dwindle due to chemical exposure, the delicate balance of food webs is disrupted, threatening biodiversity and the stability of these environments.

Shifting our focus from synthetic pigments to another prevalent component in lip products, petroleum jelly—or petrolatum—is valued for its emollient properties. This ingredient, a byproduct of oil refining, is widely used in lipsticks and glosses for its ability to create a smooth, hydrating layer on the lips, offering that sought-after glossy look and moisture barrier. However, while it may be effective as an emollient, petroleum jelly comes with serious environmental costs.

The journey of petroleum jelly begins with oil drilling, a process linked to greenhouse gas emissions, deforestation, and disruption of ecosystems. Oil extraction is energy-intensive and environmentally invasive, often leaving a legacy of pollution and habitat destruction. Furthermore, once petroleum-based products like petroleum jelly enter water systems—whether from washing off during the day or through improper disposal—they become persistent pollutants. Petroleum compounds don't break down easily, and as they accumulate in water, they begin to coat the surfaces of plants and animals.

This coating disrupts vital processes, especially for aquatic life that relies on gas exchange through their skin or gills. When plants and animals in these ecosystems are coated with these substances, their respiration and other essential functions are hindered, leading to further harm in already delicate environments. Petroleum jelly's environmental footprint stretches far beyond its immediate use, contributing to broader issues of pollution and ecosystem instability that touch both the natural world and our own lives.

What was meant to soften and protect our lips becomes a lasting pollutant, making its way through waterways and affecting countless forms of life.

The Hidden Costs of Nose Care Products

In addition to eyes and lips, I would like to shift our focus to the products we use for our noses. Products like pore strips have grown popular for their promise of visibly removing blackheads and clearing clogged pores, leaving users with that satisfying evidence of a "deep clean." However, the ingredients packed into these products tell a different story, revealing risks that extend beyond what's visible to the naked eye.

Many pore strips contain synthetic compounds like phthalates and polyethylene. Phthalates, commonly used in cosmetic products, act as plasticizers, lending flexibility and durability to the strips, making them easier to apply and ensuring they stick firmly to the skin. Yet, these same compounds are known to interfere with our body's hormonal system, as phthalates are categorized as endocrine disruptors. Their potential effects on human health are significant—prolonged exposure has been linked to reproductive health issues, developmental problems, and in some cases, even cancer. What we use to clean our pores might, in turn, be adding toxins to our bodies over time.

The environmental story doesn't end there. Once discarded, phthalates leach into soil and water, resisting natural breakdown. This resistance allows them to linger in the environment, where they continue to disrupt hormonal systems—but this time, in wildlife.

We find another problematic ingredient in pore strips—polyethylene. This plastic component is commonly used to form the adhesive layer that binds to impurities and pulls them out of the skin. While effective, polyethylene comes with a heavy environmental toll. Derived from petroleum and non-biodegradable, polyethylene becomes a lasting pollutant once discarded. Over time, it fragments into microplastics, adding to the widespread plastic pollution that is now permeating soil and air.

Many pore strips also contain preservatives, such as parabens, which prevent microbial growth. However, parabens are yet another class of chemicals known to disrupt hormonal balance in both humans and wildlife. Once parabens enter the environment through discarded products or manufacturing runoff, they can infiltrate ecosystems and interfere with the hormonal systems of wildlife, affecting species like amphibians and birds. These animals play indispensable roles, such as controlling insect populations and pollinating plants, functions critical for ecosystem balance.

The cumulative effect of these synthetic chemicals in nose care products stretches far beyond the immediate area where they are used. When these substances persist in the environment, they continue to disrupt ecosystems over long periods. Species ingesting or absorbing these chemicals often experience reduced fertility, altered behaviors, and even difficulties in finding food or escaping predators. Each disruption impacts the ecosystem, undermining biodiversity and threatening essential services like pollination and natural pest control. The persistence of these synthetic materials in nature serves as a grim reminder that even small, seemingly harmless daily habits can carry consequences that linger for decades, impacting individual organisms and entire ecosystems.

Nurturing Eyes, Nose, and Lips with Care

When we acknowledge the effects of synthetic products on our bodies and the environment, it's clear how important it is to switch to natural alternatives. Especially for sensitive areas like our eyes, nose, and lips, making this change can be incredibly beneficial. It helps us take care of our skin gently, without the harsh chemicals that can cause irritation.

Natural alternatives offer a gentle, harmonious way to support skin health. The skin around our eyes, nose, and lips is uniquely sensitive—an area that absorbs chemicals quickly and is also vulnerable to reactions. Synthetic ingredients found in conventional products can irritate and disrupt this sensitive skin, often leading to dryness, redness, and in some cases, long-term damage. Natural ingredients, on the other hand, work in synergy with the skin, offering essential nutrients without the risks associated with chemical exposure.

Natural oils, for instance, are particularly effective for these areas, providing hydration and a protective barrier against environmental stressors. Natural oils are known for their soothing properties, helping to maintain the skin's moisture balance and reduce inflammation. Plant-based extracts can further support this by calming irritation and providing antioxidants to combat daily stressors like UV rays and pollution.

When we truly appreciate nature's healing powers, we begin to understand how natural substances help us connect with the rhythms and cycles that sustain life. The delicate skin around our eyes, nose, and lips is constantly exposed to external stressors—whether it's the harsh wind, scorching sun, screen jobs or urban pollution. Natural ingredients nurture the skin without interfering with its natural defenses.

For instance, antioxidant-rich oils like argan actively combat free radicals, reducing the signs of aging around sensitive areas such as the eyes and lips. Similarly, anti-inflammatory ingredients like chamomile and calendula gently soothe irritation around the nose, particularly during allergy season or after exposure to rough weather.

Unlike synthetic solutions that often chase quick results with harsh methods, natural alternatives enhance the skin's innate resilience. They promote healing, regeneration, and balance at a cellular level, aligning with the body's natural rhythms instead of disrupting them.

But the benefits of natural products extend beyond personal care. Unlike synthetic counterparts, these are free of harmful chemicals, making them safer for everyone, including the little ones in our lives. Consider a mom, her face adorned with synthetic makeup, planting a loving kiss on her child. With every touch, trace amounts of chemicals from those products might be absorbed into the child's delicate system. Over time, these seemingly small exposures can add up, creating potential long-term concerns. Now picture the same moment, but with natural products—clean, safe, and free of toxins. If inhaled, touched, or even ingested in tiny amounts, these natural alternatives pose no harm, giving parents peace of mind and children the protection they deserve.

From an environmental perspective, shifting to natural care makes a tangible difference in reducing the environmental impact of our beauty routines. Conventional cosmetics often rely on petrochemical ingredients, synthetic fragrances, and non-biodegradable preservatives, which can linger in ecosystems long after they're washed off our skin. These ingredients disrupt wildlife and harm the environment through pollution and resource depletion in their production and disposal. Choosing natural products, on the other hand, favors ingredients like plant oils, herbal extracts, and clays—resources that are biodegradable and, when sourced responsibly, support sustainable agricultural practices. This conscious choice lessens our reliance on industrial processes, leading to a reduced ecological footprint and promoting a healthier balance with nature.

Nurturing Eyes Naturally

Switching to natural alternatives was one of the best changes I made for my skin—and it's surprisingly easy. Let me share a few of my favorite go-to methods, starting with effective natural options for caring for eyebrows and eyelids without the usual chemical-heavy products.

Castor Oil

If you're looking for a way to enhance the appearance of your eyebrows, cold pressed castor oil is perfect addition to your routine. This natural remedy has been trusted for generations to encourage hair growth gently and effectively. Packed with ricinoleic acid, castor oil nourishes hair follicles, helping to boost thickness and health over time. It also has omega-6 fatty acids and vitamin E, which keep the skin beneath the brows soft and flake-free, providing the ideal environment for healthy growth.

To use it, apply a small amount of castor oil to your brows with a cotton swab or just clean finger tips. Take a moment to gently massage; the oil works best when it's allowed to absorb overnight, so your eyebrows benefit fully from the nutrients. With daily use, you'll notice the difference in your brows' fullness and strength.

Olive Oil

The delicate skin on the eyelids benefits greatly from olive oil, a rich, natural source of antioxidants like vitamin E and polyphenols. Olive oil shields the skin from environmental stressors like UV exposure and provides lasting hydration to prevent dryness and irritation. Its anti-inflammatory qualities can also soothe puffiness and redness, making it ideal for anyone looking to reduce signs of tiredness or stress around the eyes.

Warm a few drops of olive oil between your fingers, then gently massage it onto your eyelids in circular motions. It feels wonderfully soothing, and the gentle massage promotes both absorption and relaxation. This simple routine has become a favorite in my nighttime skincare, as it leaves my eyelids feeling rejuvenated by morning.

Under-Eye Care the Natural Way

After finding natural solutions for eyebrows and eyelids, it's only natural to want a gentle approach for the delicate under-eye area as well. The skin here is so sensitive, and it's often where signs of stress, fatigue, or age start to show. Here are a few tried-and-true natural remedies that care for this delicate area and deliver real results over time.

Potato Juice

One of the simplest, most effective remedies I've come across for under-eye puffiness and dark circles is potato juice. Potatoes contain catecholase, an enzyme that's known for its ability to lighten skin, which can help reduce dark circles caused by fatigue or even genetics. Besides, the coolness of potato juice is incredibly soothing, helping to bring down any inflammation around the eyes.

To make use of this, grate a raw potato and squeeze out the juice with a cloth or strainer. Soak a cotton pad in the juice, place it over your closed eyes, and let it work for about 10-15 minutes. Afterward, rinse with cool water. Doing this regularly can make a noticeable difference, giving your under-eye area a brighter, more refreshed look.

Almond Oil

Almond oil is a fantastic natural option for anyone looking to keep the under-eye area moisturized and nourished. It's packed with vitamin E, essential fatty acids, and antioxidants, which help reduce dark circles and promote good blood circulation. Its moisturizing properties are particularly helpful in preventing the dryness that often leads to fine lines in the area.

For best results, pat a few drops of sweet almond oil around your eyes each night on clean skin. Gently massage it in circular motions to help with absorption, then leave it on overnight. This nightly ritual allows the nutrients in the oil to sink in and rejuvenate your skin as you sleep, creating a more hydrated and refreshed look by morning.

Almond Paste Application

If almond oil brings relief, then almond paste takes it a step further, offering an even richer blend of nutrients for the under-eye area. When you combine crushed almonds with milk or honey, you create a natural remedy that goes beyond hydration. Packed with biotin (vitamin B7) and minerals like manganese, this paste deeply nourishes the skin and helps maintain elasticity. It's especially beneficial for those moments when you want to reduce signs of fatigue and bring a glow back to the under-eye area.

To prepare, soak a handful of almonds overnight. In the morning, peel off the skins and grind the almonds into a fine paste using a blender or a mortar and pestle. Mix this with a bit of raw milk or honey until it's smooth and creamy. Gently apply this nourishing paste under your eyes and leave it on for about 15-20 minutes, allowing your skin to absorb the rich nutrients. Rinse it off with lukewarm water to reveal brighter, refreshed under-eyes.

These natural alternatives care for the delicate skin around your eyes and connect you to simple, effective ingredients that support your skin's health in a gentle, holistic way.

Lip Care with Natural Ingredients

Now that we've explored natural ways to care for the eyes and under-eyes, let's turn to the lips. Our lips endure exposure to sun, dry air, and the sometimes harsh ingredients in lip products. Embracing natural substances for lip care nourishes and helps maintain a natural color that many chemical-based products can dull over time.

Coriander Leaves

Starting with Coriander Leaves Paste, we find a refreshingly simple solution to brighten and restore lip color. Coriander leaves are packed with vitamins A, C, and K, which work together to gently reduce pigmentation and provide a subtle, natural glow. Regular use of coriander paste can gradually bring back the natural tone to lips affected by sun exposure, smoking, or synthetic ingredients. Plus, the antibacterial nature of coriander keeps lips free from potential infections or sores.

To make the paste, take a handful of fresh coriander leaves and grind them with a little water until smooth. Apply the paste directly to your lips, leave it on for 15-20 minutes, and then rinse with lukewarm water. With daily use, you'll start to notice a natural improvement in color and texture.

Rose Petals

Another wonderful option is rose petals—a beauty secret that's as timeless as it is effective. Beyond their fragrance, rose petals contain natural oils and sugars that provide deep hydration, making them ideal for soothing and softening chapped or cracked lips. They also offer a soft, pink tint, adding a natural flush to your lips without any artificial pigments.

To create a rose petal treatment, soak a handful of fresh rose petals in milk for a few hours to soften. Grind the soaked petals into a smooth paste and apply it to your lips, leaving it on for about 15 minutes. Gently rinse with water, and enjoy the softness and subtle color. With regular use, rose petals can keep your lips nourished and naturally tinted, bringing out their natural beauty in the most gentle way.

Sugar and Honey Scrub

A sugar and honey scrub brings the perfect blend of gentle exfoliation and deep moisture to your lips. Sugar works as a mild exfoliant, helping to slough off dry, flaky skin without irritation. Paired with honey's hydrating and healing properties, this scrub smooths and softens, giving your lips a healthy, natural glow.

To make this scrub, mix one teaspoon of sugar with half a teaspoon of honey to create a gritty paste. Gently massage it onto your lips in circular motions for one to two minutes, then rinse with lukewarm water. Follow up with a natural lip balm or oil for added hydration. Using this scrub once or twice a week keeps your lips smooth and refreshed.

Ghee

Ghee, or clarified butter, is an age-old Ayurvedic remedy treasured for its intense moisturizing abilities. Packed with essential fatty acids like omega-3s, ghee sinks into the skin, providing deep nourishment to repair dryness and cracking. Its anti-inflammatory properties also make it soothing for irritated or chapped lips, especially in colder or windy conditions.

For an intensive overnight treatment, warm a small amount of ghee and apply it directly to your lips before bed. Massage gently to encourage absorption, and leave it on overnight. By morning, your lips will feel softer and deeply hydrated, ready to take on the day.

Almond Oil

Almond oil, with its rich content of vitamin E and essential fatty acids, offers a gentle yet powerful way to keep lips moisturized. It helps repair damaged skin cells and provides lasting hydration, making it particularly useful during colder months when lips are prone to dryness and peeling.

To use almond oil, simply apply two to three drops directly onto your lips and massage until it's fully absorbed. This can become part of your daily skincare routine or be used as an overnight treatment for extra softness.

Beetroot for Lip Tinting

Following almond oil, beetroot emerges as a remarkable natural alternative for enhancing lip color. Rich in antioxidants and natural pigments, beetroot offers a range from light pink to dark pink hues, depending on how it's used. This nourishes the lips and provides them with a healthy, vibrant tint that looks effortlessly natural.

To incorporate beetroot into your lip care routine, simply grate a small piece of fresh beetroot and squeeze out the juice. Apply this juice to your lips with a cotton swab or your fingertip, allowing it to sit for about 15-20 minutes before rinsing off. For a longer-lasting tint, you can mix a few drops of beetroot juice with a carrier oil like almond oil or ghee, and leave it on overnight. Regular use will give your lips a beautiful color and keep them hydrated.

Natural Remedies for Nose Care

Now let's talk about caring for the skin around your nose. It's a delicate area that often needs a little extra attention, especially with all the exposure it gets to wind, sun, and pollution. When it comes to exfoliating and cleaning your nose, the same natural ingredients we've explored for face and body care, such as rice powder, gram flour, and masoor dal, work beautifully here too. These gentle, effective scrubs help remove dirt and dead skin without being harsh, making them perfect for this sensitive spot. You can revisit the insights and recipes from earlier chapters to incorporate these natural remedies into your nose care routine, ensuring a consistent, holistic approach to nurturing your skin. Additionally,

I want to share the following natural remedies that can effectively support the skin around your nose.

Turmeric Paste

Turmeric brings powerful anti-inflammatory and antibacterial benefits, making it an excellent choice for treating blackheads and occasional acne around the nose. Curcumin, turmeric's active compound, targets inflammation and redness, helping to soothe the skin and reduce pore blockage caused by bacteria. Additionally, turmeric naturally brightens the skin, gradually reducing pigmentation around the nose, often caused by sun exposure or lingering acne scars.

To make a turmeric paste, mix a teaspoon of turmeric powder with a few drops of water or honey until it forms a smooth paste. Apply this gently around your nose, focusing on any areas prone to blackheads or spots. Leave it on for 10 to 15 minutes, then rinse off with lukewarm water. Using this treatment two to three times a week can help keep pores clear and skin brightened over time.

Aloe Vera Gel

Aloe vera, celebrated for its soothing properties, is an ideal natural remedy for calming irritated skin around the nose—whether from allergies, sun exposure, or dryness. Its anti-inflammatory properties reduce redness and swelling, while its moisturizing effects keep the skin hydrated and prevent the flakiness that can result from cold weather or frequent nose-blowing. Additionally, aloe vera is rich in antioxidants like vitamins C and E, which not only nourish but also protect the skin from environmental damage.

To use aloe vera for nose care, extract fresh gel from an aloe vera leaf (or use store-bought pure aloe gel), and apply a thin layer directly to your nose. Massage it in gently until fully absorbed, leaving it on overnight as a calming treatment or applying it as needed throughout the day to soothe irritation.

Honey

Honey brings yet another powerful and gentle approach to keeping the skin around your nose healthy and clear. Honey is exceptional at drawing moisture into the skin, ensuring hydration in areas prone to dryness or irritation. Its humectant nature helps retain moisture, which is essential for maintaining a smooth and supple texture on the skin around the nose.

Besides hydration, honey's antibacterial properties work effectively to combat acne and prevent blackheads. It's a perfect fit for acne-prone areas, as honey can target and reduce acne-causing bacteria on the skin's surface. The natural enzymes in honey also help with gentle exfoliation, removing dead skin cells that tend to block pores and lead to blemishes. By gently sloughing off these cells, honey keeps your pores open, which is vital for preventing the formation of blackheads and maintaining a clean, healthy appearance.

To make the most of honey's benefits, apply a thin layer of raw honey to a clean nose, letting it sit for about 10-15 minutes. This simple act of self-care allows honey's enzymes to work their magic, leaving the area soft, moisturized, and refreshed. If you're looking for a bit more exfoliation, consider mixing in a small amount of cinnamon or sugar with the honey. This blend acts as a mild scrub, enhancing the exfoliation process without the harshness of synthetic alternatives. Using this treatment two to three times a week can be a gentle yet effective way to keep your nose hydrated, clear, and free from unwanted impurities.

Embracing a Natural Transition

Starting with natural alternatives for facial care can feel like a fresh start, a chance to nourish your skin without the baggage of synthetic chemicals.

But as with any change, a thoughtful approach will help you get the most out of this journey.

First, take a moment to identify what your skin truly needs. Everyone's skin is unique, and each type—whether oily, dry, sensitive, or a combination—responds differently to ingredients. For instance, if you have oily skin, you might find that certain natural oils help balance sebum production without clogging pores. Dry skin types, on the other hand, should focus on ingredients that deeply hydrate and lock in moisture. Those with sensitive skin will benefit from a more cautious approach, prioritizing soothing and gentle ingredients that don't overwhelm.

Once you have a sense of your skin's needs, start with a patch test. Even though natural ingredients are usually gentle, everyone's skin has its own quirks. A small test area—like the inside of your elbow—is a great way to check for any reaction. Wait a day or two and see how your skin responds. If there's no redness or itching, you're good to move forward. This small step is especially important when applying new products to sensitive areas like the face.

As you incorporate these new natural products, keep an eye on how your skin reacts. Some people experience a brief period of "purging," where detoxifying ingredients bring impurities to the surface. This is normal and often subsides in a few weeks, but prolonged irritation might mean a product doesn't suit your skin. For those with very sensitive skin, start with calming ingredients like aloe vera or chamomile before moving to stronger options.

Lastly, consistency and patience are your best allies in this transition. Natural products often work more gradually than their synthetic counterparts, taking time to nourish the skin on a deeper level. Stick with it, even if the results aren't immediate; over weeks or months, you'll likely notice a balanced, healthier complexion. Many find that their skin becomes more resilient with time, as natural ingredients help restore and maintain its natural balance. This steady approach lets your skin detoxify and allows it to settle into a healthier, more rooted state.

As you explore these new practices, remember that each small step brings you closer to a skincare routine that's kinder to your skin and the world around you.

Chapter 9

Neck and Décolletage – Chemicals Lurking Below the Chin

You stand in front of the mirror, carefully applying your skincare products, layer by layer. Your face glows, reflecting the hours and effort you put into keeping it healthy. But as your gaze drifts down just a bit—to your neck and the skin right below your collarbone—something feels off. The skin there tells a different story: it's a bit thinner, maybe a little drier, and, if you look closely, there's a hint of lines that don't match the rest of your reflection.

Our neck and décolletage often go unnoticed in the daily rituals that keep our face nourished and protected. This area is every bit as exposed as our face to the elements—the sun, the pollution, the stress of everyday wear and tear—but it rarely gets the same attention.

Yet it's this skin that supports us in so many subtle ways. It's the skin that carries our head high, bears the weight of necklaces and scarves, and still manages to look graceful when we hold ourselves with confidence. It stretches when we look up, turns smoothly as we nod or greet someone, and bears the weight of the many expressions we wear. And still, somehow, it tends to miss out on the care it deserves.

You, too, miss out on the care for your neck and décolletage that you deserve.

It's easy to overlook, right? We focus on making our face look youthful and vibrant, but just a few inches lower, our skin is quietly telling its own story—a story of neglect, of exposure without the comfort of creams, and of fine lines that reflect years of forgetting that this skin needs just as much care.

The irony is, while we pamper our face with expensive creams and potions, the neck and décolletage end up absorbing whatever is left—often harsh perfumes or residues from body lotions filled with chemicals we wouldn't want anywhere near sensitive skin. And you already know that many of these products do more harm than good. High-concentration alcohols, for instance, found in perfumes and sprays, can dry out and irritate this delicate skin. Ingredients like retinoids or even certain "brightening" agents can cause sensitivity and long-term damage, especially when applied without thought to sun protection.

Imagine if we shifted our attention to the neck and décolletage with the same care we give to our faces. What if, instead of using synthetic creams, we opted for gentle oils and nourishing butters made from natural ingredients? This way, we could provide the nourishment this skin needs while also helping our planet by supporting sustainable practices and reducing chemical pollution in our water and air.

In this chapter, we're going to explore that forgotten space right below your chin. You are about to make that shift. We'll explore what goes into those neck and chest products, revealing ingredients that might surprise you, and we'll look at the environmental impact of these everyday choices. Together, we'll uncover natural alternatives that are just as effective—maybe even more so—and learn simple techniques to protect and care for the skin below the chin.

Because if our body is a temple, then every part of it deserves thoughtful care, from the top of our heads to the base of our hearts.

The Hidden Chemicals in Neck and Décolletage Products

As we turn our focus to the neck and décolletage, it's important to ask: what exactly are we applying to these delicate areas each day? While we usually choose skincare products for our face with meticulous care, the products we use on our neck and chest often don't get the same level of attention or scrutiny.

This skin is thinner and has fewer oil glands, which makes it more susceptible to dryness, irritation, and early signs of aging. It's a sensitive area, and some ingredients that work well for other parts of the body can be too harsh here, potentially causing long-term issues that may go unnoticed until later.

In our daily lives, we're surrounded by advertisements that promise flawless, ageless skin.

You might have seen commercials for products that feature retinoids, claiming to smooth out wrinkles and keep the skin youthful. With all the glowing reviews and "proven" benefits, it's easy to believe that these products are exactly what our skin needs. But what often goes unsaid is how powerful these ingredients can be—and that the delicate skin on our neck and décolletage might not benefit the same way our face does.

Retinoids: The Double-Edged Sword of Anti-Aging

Retinoids are known for their ability to fight wrinkles and fine lines. They're popular in anti-aging products because they can boost collagen, making skin look firmer and smoother. But retinoids also make the skin more sensitive to sunlight. While this might be fine for parts of the face, the thinner skin on the neck can react differently.

Studies from the *Journal of Dermatological Treatment* (2020) found that retinoids, while effective, increase sensitivity to UV exposure. For areas like the neck, which might not get the same sun protection as the face, this can mean sun damage over time—exactly the opposite of what we're hoping for.

It's worth thinking twice about whether retinoids are truly the best choice for this area.

Bleaching Agents (Hydroquinone): Risky Brightening Solutions

Hydroquinone is a common ingredient in neck and décolletage creams, known for its skin-brightening properties or for 'evening out' skin tone. You may have noticed this ingredient in products from brands that focus on promoting "glow" or "radiance."

Used to even out pigmentation and reduce dark spots, it's especially popular among those looking to correct sun damage. However, hydroquinone is a powerful bleaching agent that, over time, can disrupt the skin's natural barrier and cause irritation—especially in sensitive areas.

Research published in the *American Journal of Clinical Dermatology* (2021) has shown that prolonged use of hydroquinone may lead to health risks, so much so that the EU has restricted its use in over-the-counter products. While it may initially promise smoother, more even skin, the long-term effects—particularly when used frequently on thinner skin—raise important questions about its safety. For the neck and décolletage, where the skin is more vulnerable, this ingredient can be harsh, leaving many to wonder if the short-term results are worth the potential irritation and sensitivity that come with it.

High-Concentration Alcohols: A Quick Fix with Lasting Consequences

If you've used lotions or serums on your neck that promise a "quick-drying" effect, chances are they contain high concentrations of alcohol. Alcohol is often added to skincare products for its ability to deliver a fast-absorbing, matte finish, but this comes at a cost. Alcohol-based products can strip the skin of its natural oils, leading to dryness and irritation. While this might not be a major issue for oily skin on other parts of the body, it's a different story for the neck and décolletage.

Imagine this delicate skin being exposed to alcohol day after day—without the natural oil glands needed to keep it hydrated, it can easily become dry, rough, and prone to premature aging. Instead of achieving that "smooth and firm" look, high-alcohol formulations often end up doing the opposite, accelerating the very signs of aging they claim to prevent.

In the rush for instant results, these chemicals may offer a short-lived sense of improvement, but they risk undermining the long-term health and beauty of the skin they're supposed to protect.

And when we think of our body as a temple, each choice we make for it should reflect the care and respect it deserves.

It's understandable why these ingredients are so popular. We see the promises of "quick results" and want to believe they're good for us. But the truth is, these chemicals might be doing more harm than good, especially on skin as delicate as the neck and décolletage.

There is another way, though. Natural alternatives can be just as effective without the side effects, giving this sensitive area the gentle care it needs.

While we think about what these products do to our skin, we rarely pause to consider what they're doing to the world around us. From "luxury" labels to "exotic" ingredients, the marketing behind high-end skincare paints a glamorous picture, but it often leaves out the environmental cost that comes with each jar, bottle, or spray.

Environmental Implications of High-End Skincare Products

Think of all those skincare products promising exclusive, high-performance ingredients from faraway lands. They feel special, almost magical, but every ingredient that has traveled across continents to reach your shelf carries its own invisible carbon footprint.

These words evoke images of pure, natural ingredients sourced from beautiful, faraway lands. It's easy to get swept up in the allure of a product that feels like it's been crafted just for us, with exclusive ingredients like "Moroccan argan oil" or "rare Amazonian butter." But each jar, bottle, or spray carries an environmental footprint that these glamorous labels rarely mention.

Many high-end skincare products for the neck and décolletage rely on ingredients that come from distant or ecologically sensitive areas. Take argan oil, for instance—a popular addition to many high-end products because it's known for its nourishing properties. But argan oil mostly comes from Morocco, which means it has to be transported across long distances, often using energy-intensive shipping methods that contribute significantly to carbon emissions.

A recent Life Cycle Analysis published by the *International Journal of Environmental Research* (2022) found that sourcing ingredients like argan oil and other rare plant extracts can account for 30-40% of a product's total carbon footprint, factoring in transportation, extraction, and manufacturing. So while the bottle in our hands feels like a small choice, its impact on the environment stretches far beyond our daily routine.

Take a moment to ask yourself: is this small bottle of exotic skincare truly necessary for healthy skin? And what is the cost of this health if it comes at the expense of the planet's well-being?

Then there's the impact on the land itself. Natural ingredients like shea butter and argan oil may sound eco-friendly, but high demand has led to issues with sustainability. To keep up with this demand, local ecosystems often bear the burden, with some areas facing deforestation or land conversion to make way for these "natural" resources.

A closer look at the argan oil industry in Morocco, for example, reveals some of these challenges. Studies by the Food and Agriculture Organization highlight how the rising global demand for argan oil has strained local tree populations. Argan trees are vital to the ecosystem, helping support the soil, wildlife, and local communities that depend on them. As demand increases, the pressure on these natural habitats also rises, putting local biodiversity at risk.

It doesn't stop there. Even products we don't apply directly to our skin, like perfumes and body sprays, can impact the environment in surprising ways. Many of these products contain volatile organic compounds (VOCs), which are released into the air as tiny particles. Once released, these VOCs don't just disappear—they contribute to both indoor and outdoor air pollution.

A study from the *Journal of the Air & Waste Management Association* (2021) found that VOCs in consumer products, such as perfumes and body sprays, significantly add to indoor air pollution. The effect isn't limited to personal health; it extends to broader air quality concerns. In cities already grappling with air quality issues, like Delhi, the added VOCs from household products contribute to smog formation and worsen public health concerns.

When VOCs are released, they interact with other elements in the air to create ground-level ozone—a key component of smog.

Smog doesn't cloud up the air; it contains pollutants that can irritate the respiratory system, affect visibility, and even harm crops. For cities that already deal with high pollution levels, the VOCs from skincare products, perfumes, and sprays make an already challenging situation even worse.

In Delhi, for instance, where smog often blankets the city, these everyday consumer products add to the deterioration of air quality. It's easy to overlook the role of a simple spray or lotion, but together, these choices contribute to a much larger environmental problem, one that affects not only our health but also the health of our planet.

So, while our skincare products promise luxury and beauty, it's worth remembering the hidden costs that come with them. The very products we trust to protect our skin can have far-reaching impacts, touching the air we breathe and the ecosystems that sustain us.

But there is a gentler, more mindful way to care for the neck and décolletage!

These areas deserve as much care and consideration as our face, and with natural ingredients, we can offer them just that—without the chemical load or environmental footprint. Just imagine treating your delicate skin with oils, butters, and locally sourced ingredients that nourish deeply and align with our body's natural needs. Not only can these alternatives give your skin the hydration and resilience it craves, but they also support sustainable, eco-friendly practices that benefit our environment and communities.

Going Natural – Gentle Alternatives for Neck and Décolletage Care

You might remember watching your grandmother warm up a little oil and massage it onto her face, arms, and neck before bed. She'd rely on simple things, like coconut oil or almond oil, with no fancy names or luxury packaging. And somehow, her skin stayed soft and smooth without needing a lineup of high-end skincare. The idea of slathering our skin with creams and serums full of complex ingredients is relatively new. In India, skincare has always been about using what's around us, nurturing the skin with simple, natural ingredients that not only keep us healthy but respect our surroundings too.

In traditional Indian skincare, oils, herbs, and butters were valued not only for their effectiveness but for how they align with the idea of *ahimsa*, or non-violence. It's a belief that caring for yourself shouldn't harm the environment. These natural oils and butters are kind to both the skin and the planet—a way of taking care of ourselves that feels connected to something larger.

Natural Oils for Nourishment and Hydration

For centuries, Indian households have turned to simple oils like almond, coconut, mustard and sesame for skin care. These oils are still some of the best choices for sensitive areas like the neck, offering deep hydration without clogging or irritating the skin. They're gentle, they're effective, and best of all, they're sustainable.

Almond Oil: Rich in Vitamin E and essential fatty acids, almond oil is a wonderful match for the delicate skin on the neck. Its nourishing properties make it gentle and soothing, ideal for areas that need a bit of extra care. After a shower, try warming a few drops of almond oil in your hands and gently massage it into your neck in upward motions. This locks in moisture, keeping the skin soft and hydrated. If you're looking for a nighttime treat, you can even mix almond oil with a little aloe vera gel to keep the skin supple and fresh as you sleep.

Argan Oil: Known as "liquid gold," argan oil is deeply hydrating and works wonders for promoting elasticity. To use, simply warm a few drops between your palms and massage it in light, upward strokes along the neck and décolletage. This not only hydrates but also boosts circulation, which helps prevent sagging. Argan oil's lightweight feel makes it easy to apply daily without any greasiness, so you can enjoy its benefits without feeling weighed down.

Butters for Deep Moisture and Protection

For days when your skin feels especially dry, natural butters like shea and cocoa can offer extra moisture and a protective barrier. Unlike lotions with artificial emollients, these butters are packed with vitamins and fatty acids that work harmoniously with the skin.

Shea Butter: High in vitamins A and E, shea butter is a powerful moisturizer that forms a natural barrier against environmental stressors. It's also known for its anti-inflammatory properties, which help soothe sensitive skin. To ensure sustainability, try to choose shea butter from sources that support local farmers and protect biodiversity. To apply, warm a small amount between your fingers and gently massage it into the neck, paying attention to areas where fine lines tend to develop. Shea butter's thick consistency creates a lasting shield, keeping skin hydrated throughout the day.

Cocoa Butter: Rich in antioxidants, cocoa butter is another great option for protecting the skin and improving elasticity. Known for its subtle, natural fragrance and smooth texture, cocoa butter can be used as a massage cream for the neck, especially in areas prone to fine lines. A simple Indian nuska or remedy is to slightly warm cocoa butter before application; this allows it to spread more easily and absorb better. Massage it into the skin, focusing on upward strokes that encourage firmness.

Locally Sourced Ingredients for a Sustainable Routine

Ingredients that grow close to home, like coconut and sesame oil, are fantastic for the skin and don't come with the same transportation emissions as imported ingredients. In India, sesame oil has long been used for its nourishing and protective qualities, especially during the winter when skin tends to be drier.

Sesame Oil: Known in Ayurvedic practices as a "warming oil," sesame oil is deeply moisturizing and helps to lock in hydration. Its rich nutrient profile makes it ideal for sensitive areas like the neck, as it forms a natural barrier that protects against dryness and environmental stress. Apply a small amount to the neck and décolletage, and let it absorb naturally. Its earthy fragrance is both grounding and gentle, making it a simple, effective addition to your routine.

Mustard Oil: Mustard oil is another excellent locally sourced option, celebrated for its intense moisturizing properties and protective benefits. Rich in omega-3 and omega-6 fatty acids, as well as antioxidants like vitamin E, mustard oil can be particularly effective during the dry winter months. It is known to stimulate circulation, which can help to revitalize and warm the skin, making it a popular choice for massages and body oils. When applied to the skin, it forms a revitalizing layer that hydrates and can protect against external pollutants. To use, warm the oil slightly and massage gently onto the skin, allowing its invigorating properties to nourish deeply.

Coconut Oil: Coconut oil is another widely available and sustainable option. Known for its hydrating properties, it's a versatile choice that suits most skin types. A light massage with coconut oil can keep the neck skin soft and resilient. You can even add a few drops of essential oil, like lavender or rose, to enhance the experience.

Choosing these natural, locally sourced alternatives isn't just a choice for your skin; it's a choice for the planet. These ingredients don't carry the same hidden costs as high-end luxury items, and they honor a slower, more thoughtful approach to beauty—one that treats both your skin and the environment with respect, the kind you know that both you and Mother Earth deserve.

But how we apply these oils and butters matters just as much as what we're using.

A little mindfulness in your skincare routine can make all the difference, helping these natural ingredients work their best without wastage. Small adjustments to how and when you apply them can maximize their benefits, turning each application into a simple ritual of care.

Application Tips for Maximum Benefit

Warm the Oils for Better Absorption

Warming oils before applying can help them penetrate the skin more deeply, enhancing hydration and maximizing their nourishing effects. Think of it like warming a compress; the gentle heat allows the oils to sink in more effectively, especially on the neck and décolletage, where skin can be prone to dryness.

To do this, pour a few drops of oil into your palms and rub them together to generate warmth. Then, gently press your hands onto your neck, using upward strokes from your collarbone to your jawline. This simple step can make the oil feel richer and more comforting, without needing more product than a few drops. Not only does this prevent wastage, but it also helps you experience the full soothing benefits of these oils.

Massage Techniques to Boost Circulation

In Indian traditions, massage is a cherished part of self-care, believed to not only nourish the body but also awaken the senses and promote overall wellness. By incorporating gentle massage techniques, you can encourage better circulation in the neck area, giving the skin a healthy glow and helping reduce any puffiness.

For a quick massage, start by placing your hands at the base of your neck and using slow, circular motions to press upwards toward your jawline. Think of it as gently "lifting" your skin, avoiding any downward pressure. These circular movements stimulate blood flow, which in turn helps the skin absorb the oils and butters more effectively. It's a small, calming step that can make a noticeable difference in how your skin looks and feels.

Layering for Extra Hydration and Protection

For those with drier or aging skin, layering oils, and butters can provide an added level of moisture. Begin with a lighter oil, like almond or argan, and then seal it with a richer butter, such as shea. This layering technique works much like locking moisture into a soil bed; the initial oil penetrates deeply, while the thicker butter acts as a barrier to keep everything in place.

As with any ritual, moderation is key. You don't need much product—just a few drops of oil and a dab of butter—to keep your skin soft and hydrated. This approach not only conserves your product but also respects the idea of minimalism in skincare, avoiding the excess that so often leads to waste.

Timing for Best Absorption

Timing can be everything in skincare, and applying natural oils and butters at night is one of the best ways to support your skin's natural repair processes. Nighttime is when the skin goes into recovery mode, working to repair damage from the day. By nourishing it at this time, you can enhance the effects of these natural ingredients, allowing them to work more deeply as you sleep.

Simply massage a bit of oil or butter onto your neck and décolletage as part of your evening routine, letting it absorb slowly overnight. This is particularly effective in dry seasons when the skin needs that extra layer of moisture. It's a simple habit, but one that can make your skincare feel even more rewarding, knowing that each night you're giving your skin the best conditions to heal and renew.

As you stand in front of the mirror each day, you now have a choice—a choice to extend the same care and attention you give to your face down to the skin that supports it. The neck and décolletage are a part of you, exposed to the same elements, holding up the weight of each day, and reflecting your grace and strength with every move. When you start treating this skin with the same thoughtfulness you bring to your facial care, it begins to tell a story of care and renewal, mirroring the health and vitality you've carefully nurtured.

In embracing these natural, gentle practices, you're supporting your skin's health while also stepping toward a life that honors simplicity rooted living, and connection. You're choosing oils and butters over chemicals, small rituals over quick fixes, and a deeper awareness of how your choices echo beyond the mirror. So, as you finish your skincare routine, look back at your reflection and know that every part of you, from your face down to your heart, is receiving the thoughtful care it deserves—the thoughtful care *you* deserve.

Chapter 10

Hand and Underarm Care – Handling with Care

"The human hand is a tool of tools."

— Aristotle

Our hands are remarkable, aren't they?

They hold memories and responsibilities, bearing the marks of all they've carried. They've held onto loved ones, gripped tightly in moments of excitement, steadied us through challenges, and offered comfort in times of need. Maybe they remind you of your mother's hands, weathered but gentle, or of the tiny hand of a child wrapped around your finger. Our hands bear the weight of everyday life and hold the stories of who we are, often without thanks.

And yet, think about all the things we expose them to each day. A quick pump of sanitizer, a layer of lotion, and a swipe of deodorant as we get ready. It's routine—so automatic we hardly give it a second thought. But each of these products, layered on day after day, isn't just sitting on the surface. They're absorbed into the skin, introducing chemicals meant to kill germs, block sweat, or add fragrance. Chemicals that might seem harmless but, over time, may tell a different story.

We're so used to these products promising cleanliness, freshness, and protection that it's easy to miss the hidden cost. Beneath that layer of lotion or spritz of deodorant lies a mix of ingredients that can irritate, dry out, or disrupt the body's natural balance. And it doesn't stop there—with each wash, these chemicals rinse down our drains and eventually seep into the soil and water around us, impacting more than we can see.

Imagine a different way—a way of caring for your hands and underarms that respects both your body and the world around you. Imagine using natural, gentle alternatives that nourish rather than mask, that work with your body's needs, and that honor the planet.

Because if our hands carry so much for us, then they deserve a kind of care that carries something meaningful in return.

The Chemical Handshake

Every day, we see advertisements filled with promises of "24-hour protection" and "99.9% germ kill." Brands like *Dettol* and *Dove* assure us that their hand sanitizers, soaps, and deodorants will keep us safe, clean, and fresh. It's hard not to be drawn in—especially when these words are associated with the familiar sense of cleanliness and confidence. But behind these appealing claims lies an ingredient list that's less talked about. In products we use on sensitive areas like our hands and underarms, what's left out of the ads may be just as important as what's included.

Our skin, especially in places as delicate as our hands and underarms, is constantly absorbing what we apply. And some of the chemicals in these everyday products have effects that go beyond just their antibacterial or deodorizing abilities.

Triclosan in Hand Sanitizers and Soaps

Triclosan is a common antibacterial agent you'll find in many hand sanitizers and soaps, particularly those that promise to kill germs instantly. In India, where concerns over hygiene are high, triclosan-based products have become household staples. But while triclosan does kill bacteria, it may be doing more than we bargained for.

Studies published in *The Indian Journal of Medical Research* (2021) reveal that prolonged exposure to triclosan can interfere with hormone balance, potentially disrupting our body's endocrine system. Over time, this disruption can lead to health issues that affect everything from energy levels to stress responses.

Additionally, triclosan's heavy use in soaps and sanitizers has contributed to bacterial resistance—a growing issue worldwide.

Ironically, in our effort to keep bacteria at bay, we may be giving rise to bacteria that are more resistant to antibiotics, which affects not just individual health but public health as a whole. Although triclosan is still widely available in India, awareness of these risks is prompting some to reconsider their reliance on antibacterial soaps.

Aluminum Compounds in Antiperspirants

Another common ingredient to think about is aluminum, which is found in most antiperspirants and works to block sweat. For many of us, especially in India's warm, humid climate, antiperspirants have become a necessity. But aluminum compounds do more than just keep us dry—they have raised concerns about their potential impact on health.

Research from The Indian Dermatology Online Journal (2020) indicates that long-term exposure to aluminum may cause changes in breast tissue. While studies are still ongoing, it's important to consider the potential risks of aluminum exposure, particularly for those who use antiperspirants every day.

Aside from personal health, aluminum compounds can impact the environment. When they wash off during showers, they enter our waterways and soils, leading to acidification. This change in soil chemistry makes it more difficult for plants to absorb nutrients, which ultimately affects the entire ecosystem, including both plants and animals. In rural areas where agriculture relies on healthy soil, the widespread use of aluminum becomes a significant ecological and personal concern.

Artificial Fragrances in Lotions and Deodorants

Then there are the artificial fragrances, often labeled simply as *"parfum"* in ingredient lists. These fragrances give products their signature scent, masking odors and leaving us with a sense of freshness. However, they often contain phthalates, a class of chemicals known for extending fragrance but with a hidden downside: they can disrupt hormonal function. According to studies published in *The Indian Journal of Public Health* (2022), prolonged exposure to phthalates has been linked to hormonal imbalances, which can affect reproductive health.

Popular scented products add appealing fragrances to our daily routines. However, this refreshing smell comes with a hidden cost. These fragrances may not only linger on our skin but could also impact our body's internal systems in unseen ways, making it essential to look into what exactly lies beneath the scent.

Ecosystem Impact of Hand and Underarm Care Products

The effects of these products don't end with us. Every time we wash our hands or rinse off deodorant, small amounts of these chemicals go down the drain, entering our waterways and soils. They don't simply disappear. Instead, they continue their journey into rivers, fields, and farmlands, affecting the ecosystems that support agriculture and biodiversity.

With each rinse, these ingredients make their way into our soil and water, causing effects that extend far beyond our homes and bathroom routines.

Think about aluminum, a common ingredient in antiperspirants that prevents sweating by blocking sweat production. When aluminum compounds are washed off in the shower, they accumulate in the soil over time, gradually changing their composition. This process, called soil acidification, makes soil less fertile and disrupts plant growth.

Studies published in *The Indian Journal of Agricultural Sciences* (2021) highlight that high aluminum levels in soil can interfere with plants' ability to absorb nutrients. Staple crops like wheat and rice, which need a balanced soil environment to grow well, are especially affected, leading to lower yields and reduced resilience of these plants.

This buildup creates a chain reaction. When crops struggle, so do the farmers who rely on these harvests. As yields decrease and crop quality is compromised, both the food supply and the livelihood of farming communities are impacted. What begins as a single ingredient in our deodorant can ultimately affect entire ecosystems, from the soil itself to the people and animals who depend on it.

Triclosan, another ingredient, finds its way into the soil through a different route. Waste treatment facilities often repurpose sewage sludge as fertilizer for fields. While this may seem like an efficient solution, it unintentionally introduces chemicals like triclosan into agricultural soil. Research from *The Indian Journal of Environmental Health* (2022) shows that triclosan can interfere with photosynthesis and restrict root growth in plants, which in turn reduces crop productivity. Crops absorb these chemicals, leading to lower yields and potentially affecting food quality.

The impact doesn't stop at plants. Herbivores and other animals that rely on these crops consume the chemicals along with the plants, which can affect their health and disrupt local food chains. For rural communities that rely on agriculture for their livelihood, lower crop yields can be a tough challenge, affecting everyday life and local economies. It's interesting how the products we use to stay clean and fresh can actually impact the communities that sustain us.

Besides the products we use on our skin, think about the scents that linger the air. Artificial fragrances in lotions, deodorants, and sprays contain volatile organic compounds, or VOCs, which are released as tiny particles. These VOCs contribute to ground-level ozone, one of the main components of smog. In areas that already struggle with high pollution levels, VOCs add another layer of impact, especially on air quality.

Research from The Indian Council of Medical Research (ICMR) shows that VOCs from common products are linked to respiratory health problems, like asthma and allergies, especially in crowded urban areas. Smog affects visibility, harms crop yields, and irritates the respiratory systems of both people and animals. With each application of a fragranced product, tiny particles linger, gradually influencing the quality of the air we all breathe.

The impact of these daily products on our ecosystems is easy to overlook, but by understanding the full effect of their ingredients, we begin to see why mindful choices matter.

Natural Solutions for Everyday Care

When it comes to caring for sensitive areas like our hands and underarms, there's a simpler way to meet our needs—natural alternatives that protect our skin while being gentle with the environment. Imagine replacing harsh chemicals with ingredients like coconut oil, alum, and baking soda, which have been trusted in households for generations. These are accessible, effective, and kind to both our bodies and the world around us.

For hand and underarm care, natural ingredients can offer benefits without the hidden costs. They allow us to nourish and protect our skin while supporting a healthier, more balanced planet.

Beeswax: Beeswax is a natural substance produced by honeybees. It's commonly available at local health stores or online and forms a light protective barrier over the skin, locking in moisture while allowing it to breathe. When mixed with antibacterial herbs like neem or turmeric, beeswax makes an excellent base for a hand cream. For a simple DIY hand cream, combine beeswax, coconut oil, and a few drops of neem oil to create a soothing, chemical-free moisturizer that hydrates and protects the skin from germs.

Alum: Alum, known as “fitkari” in many households, is a traditional remedy often used as a natural deodorant. It neutralizes odor-causing bacteria without blocking sweat, helping the body stay cool and balanced. Alum is affordable, widely available in local markets and general stores, and can be paired with coconut oil to create an effective underarm solution that respects your skin’s natural state. This combination provides gentle, long-lasting freshness without introducing harsh chemicals.

Baking Soda: Baking soda is another natural option for underarm care. It helps balance the skin’s pH, reducing odor without causing irritation. Widely available in most grocery stores, baking soda can be used on its own or mixed with coconut oil for a smoother application. This simple, affordable ingredient has been relied upon for years as an effective, natural way to manage odor without affecting the body’s natural processes.

Sandalwood: Sandalwood has been used in Indian skincare for centuries for its calming aroma and cooling effect on the skin. It can be applied as a paste or oil, offering a subtle, natural scent. A small amount under the arms keeps the skin cool and refreshed. Sandalwood powder or oil is easily found in local beauty stores or markets, particularly those specializing in Ayurvedic products.

Orange Peel Powder: Orange peel powder is an excellent natural exfoliant that revitalizes the skin and combats body odor. Its high vitamin C and antioxidant content helps remove dead skin cells and impurities, which can contribute to unpleasant smells. By gently scrubbing your body with a mixture of orange peel powder and water, you can cleanse the skin, unclog pores, and leave behind a fresh, citrusy scent. The natural astringent properties of orange peel also help regulate excess oil, making it particularly useful for sweat-prone areas such as the underarms. Regular use of this scrub brightens and smoothens the skin, giving it a healthy glow.

Rosewater: Rosewater is a refreshing, gentle option for fragrance. It offers a light, natural scent without the synthetic additives in most perfumes. Rosewater can be spritzed on the skin or dabbed onto pulse points for a clean, cooling fragrance. It's widely available in beauty stores and pharmacies and can also be made at home by simmering fresh rose petals in water. Rosewater is light on sensitive skin and provides a pleasant scent that doesn't overpower.

Lemon Peels: Lemon peels are rich in citric acid and can be used for effective underarm and arm care. Soaking lemon peels in a bucket of water for 30 minutes before taking a bath creates an infusion that acts as a natural deodorizer and skin lightener. This method helps eliminate odor-causing bacteria while gently exfoliating the skin and promoting an even skin tone. The citric acid in lemon peels assists in breaking down dead skin cells, making it beneficial for those with darkened or rough underarm skin. The refreshing scent of lemon also leaves your skin feeling rejuvenated and fresh throughout the day.

These simple alternatives allow us to care for our hands and underarms in a way that respects both our skin and the environment.

Each ingredient serves a purpose without relying on artificial chemicals, bringing a sense of balance and thoughtfulness to our routines.

Transition Tips for Lasting Benefits

Switching to natural alternatives doesn't need to happen overnight. Transitioning can be gradual, allowing you to explore these options at your own pace and find what works best for your body. Here are some practical steps to make the switch smooth, enjoyable, and long-lasting.

Try DIY First

Starting with simple, homemade options can be a great way to ease into natural care.

For example, mixing alum with coconut oil creates a gentle deodorant that neutralizes odor-causing bacteria without blocking sweat. Similarly, a neem-based hand balm made with coconut oil and a hint of beeswax can provide hydration and antibacterial benefits. By creating these remedies at home, you can test how your skin responds without the commitment of store-bought products. Plus, DIY solutions honor traditional "nuske," or home remedies, passed down through generations—methods that our elders trusted for their simplicity and effectiveness.

Allow Time for Adjustment

Switching to natural products may feel different at first. Unlike synthetic formulas, natural products work with your body's natural rhythms, which might take some time to adjust. For instance, a natural deodorant won't block sweat but will help manage odor. It's normal to experience a transition period as your body adapts to the change. Give it a few weeks, allowing your skin and body to find their natural balance. This patience pays off, as you'll soon notice that these gentle alternatives provide a fresher, healthier experience without the heavy layers of chemicals.

Embrace Minimalism

With natural products, simplicity is key. You'll find that a little goes a long way. Instead of layering on multiple products, try focusing on the essentials and applying small amounts. Like, a few drops of coconut oil or a small amount of beeswax balm can provide lasting hydration.

Embracing this simplicity not only reduces product waste but also brings a sense of calm to your routine.

Using fewer products benefits both your wallet and the planet, creating a balanced approach that aligns with sustainable living.

Making the switch to natural care doesn't transform your routine; it encourages a mindset of mindfulness. By approaching skincare with a focus on simplicity and patience, you'll experience benefits that extend beyond your skin—supporting your well-being and the health of the world around you.

As you look down at your hands, notice all they carry—the gestures of care, the strength in each small act, and the warmth they share with others. These hands, along with every part of your body, deserve the same gentleness and thoughtfulness that you extend to the people around you.

Caring for your hands and underarms with natural ingredients isn't merely a change in routine; it's an acknowledgment of their enduring value. Embracing ingredients like alum, sandalwood, and coconut oil connects you to a long-standing tradition of care—one that respects purity and values our relationship with the earth. Each small choice, from a soothing balm to a refreshing rosewater mist, becomes a meaningful step toward balance—a balance that cares for both your health and the world around you.

Our hands, which have carried so much for us, deserve this thoughtful care. When we choose simplicity, patience, and mindfulness, self-care transforms into a quiet, powerful act of respect. With each gentle step, we're honoring the parts of ourselves that carry us through life, and, in doing so, we honor the world that supports us.

Chapter 11

Leg Care – From Thighs to Toes

You run the water, reach for the shaving cream, and begin the familiar routine. A soft lather forms as you glide the razor along your skin, revealing a smoothness that feels instantly satisfying. Maybe it's for a night out, a special event, or just the feeling of being fresh and prepared. Or perhaps it's a hot day, and you slip on sandals, catching sight of your feet. A quick rub of foot cream seems to be all they need. And then there are those rushed mornings, standing in the shower, following the same steps you could do with your eyes closed: shave, rinse, moisturize.

These small rituals are part of getting ready, part of feeling our best. Each swipe and lather promises smooth, soft skin, and a quick fix in the name of care. But beneath the surface, these products offer more than just a feeling. Shaving foams, foot creams, moisturizers—all promising fresh, soft skin but often carrying hidden ingredients that linger long after that quick fix has faded.

And with everything they endure, don't our legs deserve more?

Our legs carry us through endless steps, long days, uphill climbs, and uneven paths, bearing the weight of everything we take on without complaint. Yet, despite all they do, they're often left with quick-fix products that offer a temporary feel of care without lasting support. Modern leg care products have evolved for convenience and effectiveness, but the very ingredients that offer smooth shaves and lasting moisture may come with unseen costs.

What's inside these products goes beyond our skin, impacting our health and the world around us.

The Chemical Coverage

In today's leg care products—whether for shaving, moisturizing, or foot care—synthetic chemicals are added to make the process faster and the results more satisfying. These ingredients help shaving creams create a thick lather, keep moisturizers fresh, and give foot creams their antifungal power. But these benefits come with hidden costs, affecting both our health and the environment around us.

Let's look closely at the common chemicals found in these products, understanding their role, their impact, and why a quick fix might not always be the best solution for lasting care for everything - thighs to toes.

Parabens in Moisturizers

Moisturizers often contain parabens, a group of preservatives added to prevent bacterial growth and extend shelf life. On the surface, they seem helpful; after all, no one wants a moisturizer that spoils quickly. But parabens don't come without concerns.

Studies from *The Journal of Applied Toxicology* (2022) show that parabens can interfere with hormone balance in the body. When used regularly, they can disrupt endocrine functions, potentially impacting reproductive health over time. Parabens are commonly listed on ingredient labels as methylparaben, ethylparaben, and butylparaben, so keeping an eye out for these names is a small yet effective step for anyone wanting to limit exposure to these chemicals.

While the intent behind parabens is to keep products safe, their effects on our bodies raise questions about whether this trade-off is truly worth it.

Synthetic Fragrances in Leg and Foot Creams

Many leg and foot creams include synthetic fragrances to create a pleasing scent. But beneath that refreshing smell lies a blend of chemicals, often including phthalates. Phthalates are known for their ability to extend the life of fragrances, but they've also been shown to interfere with hormone function.

According to *The Environmental Health Perspectives Journal* (2021), synthetic fragrances release volatile organic compounds (VOCs) that can impact indoor air quality. These VOCs don't simply disappear—they linger in enclosed spaces like bathrooms, contributing to indoor air pollution. Health studies have linked prolonged VOC exposure to respiratory issues, and even minor changes in mood and focus.

So while the scent may be appealing, the chemicals behind it can have subtle, lasting effects that go beyond a simple fragrance.

Propellants in Aerosol Shaving Creams

Aerosol shaving creams often use propellants like isobutane and propane to create a fine spray that's easy to apply. These propellants offer convenience but bring with them another layer of health and environmental concerns.

When used in small, enclosed spaces like bathrooms, these propellants release VOCs that increase indoor air pollution. The *Indian Council of Medical Research* (2023) found that regular use of aerosol sprays can lead to VOC buildup, which can irritate the respiratory tract and, for those with asthma or sensitivities, worsen symptoms over time. Beyond indoor air quality, these aerosol propellants contribute to the release of hydrocarbons into the atmosphere, affecting both the air we breathe and the environment we live in.

The quick spray from an aerosol can may seem like a small thing, but its impact is anything but.

Triclosan in Antifungal Foot Creams

Triclosan is a common ingredient in foot creams due to its antibacterial and antifungal properties. In warm climates, where people often wear closed shoes and turn to antifungal foot creams for relief, triclosan provides quick and effective results. But the widespread use of triclosan has raised significant concerns over its long-term effects.

Studies from *The Journal of Environmental Sciences* (2022) indicate that triclosan contributes to antimicrobial resistance, meaning that bacteria exposed to it over time can become resistant to treatment. When these products are washed down the drain, triclosan enters waterways, disrupting microbial ecosystems essential for maintaining environmental balance. In both soil and water, it encourages the growth of resistant bacterial strains, posing a risk to plants, animals, and ultimately, human health.

In areas where warm climates lead to frequent use of foot creams, triclosan's impact extends much beyond individual health, seeping into our water and soil and affecting ecosystems. What starts as a single ingredient in our leg care products extends outward, impacting the environment in ways we might not expect.

The Chain Reaction in Environment

The environmental footprint of our leg care products doesn't end with personal use. Many of the chemicals we apply to our skin—parabens, propellants, and artificial fragrances—travel beyond us, entering the air, soil, and water that sustain life. Over time, these ingredients contribute to pollution, affecting everything from indoor air quality to the health of ecosystems we rely on.

When we use aerosol shaving foams or sprays, for example, propellants like isobutane and propane release volatile organic compounds, or VOCs, into the air. In enclosed spaces like bathrooms, these VOCs accumulate, gradually affecting indoor air quality. The *Indian Council of Medical Research* (2023) found that frequent exposure to VOCs can increase respiratory issues, especially for those with asthma or sensitivities, turning a quick morning shave into a subtle but ongoing source of air pollution within our own homes.

But the impact of these propellants extends beyond our homes. Many aerosol products contain hydrofluorocarbons (HFCs), which, once released, rise into the atmosphere and contribute to ozone layer depletion. The *World Health Organization* (2023) has reported that emissions from HFCs continue to thin the ozone layer, reducing its ability to block harmful UV rays from reaching the Earth. This increase in UV radiation doesn't just affect us by raising the risk of skin cancer; it also disrupts delicate ecosystems, from plant life sensitive to sunlight to aquatic organisms that rely on stable light levels for survival. Each time we spray a shaving foam or foot deodorant, we're adding a bit more strain to an environment already balancing so many demands.

Meanwhile, antifungal chemicals like triclosan, commonly found in foot creams, introduce another set of concerns. These ingredients may help prevent infections, but once they're washed down the drain, they enter water treatment systems, eventually making their way into agricultural soils. Research from *The Indian Journal of Environmental Health* (2022) shows that chemicals like triclosan disrupt the natural balance of microorganisms in soil. These microbes play a critical role in keeping soil healthy and fertile, breaking down organic matter, and cycling nutrients that plants need to grow. When triclosan and similar compounds accumulate in soil, they interfere with these processes, leading to soils that are less productive and plants that struggle to thrive.

This disruption in soil health doesn't just affect plants. Microbes are the foundation of complex food chains, and their absence or imbalance can have far-reaching effects that impact larger animals, insects, and eventually humans. The overuse of antifungal chemicals has contributed to a concerning rise in antimicrobial resistance, as bacteria and fungi adapt to withstand these compounds. This makes it harder to control microbial growth in both natural and agricultural settings, adding yet another layer of complexity to an already delicate ecosystem.

With each product we use in our daily routines, we're affecting environments beyond our immediate surroundings. It's easy to think of our leg care as a personal choice, but the chemicals we apply and rinse away can impact the health of soil, air, and water in ways that last far beyond a single use. Understanding these broader effects helps us see why mindful choices matter, not only for our own health but for the world that supports us.

Herbal and Plant-Based Alternatives

For generations, traditional ingredients have been trusted to care for skin gently, offering natural benefits without the synthetic additives so common today. When it comes to cleansing the legs, there's no need for anything overly specialized. The same options discussed for body cleansing—like rice powder, besan, masoor dal, or multani mitti—work beautifully, offering a thorough clean and gentle exfoliation. These versatile natural cleansers make it easy to extend your skincare routine to your legs without any additional fuss, keeping the process simple, effective, and sustainable. Elders often relied on simple, natural remedies—coconut oil, aloe vera, and even homemade scrubs—not only because they worked, but because they kept things pure and close to nature.

Let's explore these natural ingredients that remain effective today, allowing us to honor both our bodies and the environment.

Coconut Oil

Coconut oil is well-loved for its deep hydrating qualities, a simple remedy known for keeping skin soft and resilient. After a shower, when the skin is still slightly damp, applying a small amount of coconut oil creates a natural barrier that locks in moisture, keeping the skin supple. The oil forms a protective layer that doesn't clog pores or leave the skin feeling heavy. Coconut oil is gentle, easy to store, and widely available, making it an accessible option that reduces the need for chemical-laden lotions. Its ease of use has made it a staple in many homes, a reliable moisturizer that's as kind to the skin as it is to the planet. One of the best ways to remove hair is to apply a layer of oil, or oil mixed with water, before shaving. This method prevents the skin from drying out and makes the process quick too.

Aloe Vera

Aloe vera, a plant known for its soothing and cooling properties, is a natural choice for irritated or freshly shaved skin. Its anti-inflammatory effects make it especially helpful for calming any redness or razor burn. After shaving, a light layer of aloe vera gel can calm the skin while adding a gentle touch of hydration. Many people keep an aloe vera plant in their homes, breaking off a leaf as needed to apply the fresh gel directly to the skin. This simple, sustainable source of hydration feels refreshing and cool, a natural way to nurture skin without adding unnecessary ingredients.

Homemade Sugar Scrubs

For gentle exfoliation, sugar scrubs offer a way to remove dead skin without the harshness of store-bought scrubs. Unlike synthetic scrubs containing plastic microbeads, a homemade sugar scrub is safe for the environment and leaves the skin smooth. A basic recipe combines sugar with a carrier oil, like coconut or olive oil, with an optional few drops of essential oil for fragrance—lavender or peppermint work well. This weekly ritual not only refreshes the skin but also eliminates the need for plastic-based products, helping keep waterways free of microplastic pollution.

Neem Oil

Neem oil, an age-old solution for skin health, is valued for its antifungal properties, making it perfect for foot care. Just a few drops massaged into clean feet, especially between the toes, can help prevent fungal growth. Neem oil respects the skin's natural state, working gently without promoting resistance, unlike stronger chemical antifungals. It's easy to find in health stores and has a distinct, earthy fragrance that feels grounding, reminding us of the effectiveness of simple, natural remedies. This humble ingredient serves as a powerful alternative to chemical-laden foot creams, supporting both healthy skin and environmental well-being.

Each of these natural alternatives offers a way to care for our skin in a way that feels balanced and respectful, using ingredients that align with our bodies rather than overpower them. They serve as a reminder that effective care can be simple, honoring the same approaches that generations before us trusted.

Incorporating natural leg and foot care into your routine can feel like reconnecting with mindful, time-tested practices. These small changes go beyond replacing products, creating moments that benefit your skin and the environment. Here are practical tips to make the most of these natural ingredients and turn them into lasting habits.

Best Times for Application

After Showering: Applying natural oils like coconut oil or aloe vera gel right after a shower helps lock in moisture. When skin is slightly damp, it absorbs oils more easily, allowing hydration to sink deeply without feeling greasy. A thin layer of coconut oil keeps the skin on your legs soft and nourished throughout the day, while aloe vera, with its cooling properties, is ideal for calming freshly shaved skin and adding gentle moisture that feels light and clean.

Before Bed: Bedtime is the perfect opportunity to apply neem oil or a bit of coconut oil to your feet. Overnight, these oils soften dry, rough skin and help prevent cracked heels. Neem oil, with its natural antifungal qualities, offers added protection, making it a useful addition to your routine, especially in warm weather when closed shoes are worn frequently.

Routine Suggestions

Weekly Exfoliation: A simple sugar scrub, used once a week, provides gentle exfoliation, removing dead skin and keeping legs and feet smooth. Combining sugar with coconut or olive oil and a few drops of essential oil for fragrance creates an eco-friendly scrub, replacing commercial exfoliants. This option benefits both your skin and the environment, avoiding the plastic microbeads found in many store-bought scrubs, which can contribute to water pollution.

Consistent Moisturizing: Daily use of coconut oil on both legs and feet, especially during dry seasons, provides lasting hydration. Its natural properties keep skin supple without relying on heavy lotions. This habit keeps your skin hydrated with minimal products, reducing the need for chemical-based options and cutting down on packaging waste.

Nature's best moisturizers are the oils it provides. Light or thin oils like coconut can be applied throughout the year. However, in winter, thicker oils such as sesame, olive, mustard, and castor are best for keeping the skin nourished.

Environmental Considerations

Using natural products brings advantages beyond personal care. Oils, scrubs, and homemade treatments come with minimal packaging compared to pre-packaged, synthetic products, which often use single-use plastic containers. Choosing natural alternatives reduces plastic waste and avoids the environmental impact of packaging production and disposal.

By eliminating synthetic fragrances and aerosol sprays, you avoid indoor air pollution from VOCs, supporting cleaner air in your home. These natural products support both skin health and a healthier indoor environment, benefiting everyone in your household.

Each of these practices builds a routine that values thoughtful, lasting care over quick fixes. Choosing these natural options creates habits that reflect a commitment to personal well-being and environmental awareness. With each daily ritual, there's an opportunity to care for both your body and the world in ways that feel balanced and grounded.

Our legs and feet are with us through every step, supporting us without question, no matter the terrain or distance. They bear the weight of our bodies, our days, and our journeys, moving us forward while asking so little in return. Yet, it's easy to overlook the quiet strength they provide, often giving them quick fixes instead of the care they truly deserve.

Each time we choose gentle, mindful products, we honor the parts of us that work hardest, offering them the same care they've shown us day in and day out. So, as you finish these daily rituals, take a moment to appreciate the strength and resilience of your legs and feet. Notice the comfort and lightness that natural care brings, and know that each thoughtful choice is a step toward a more rooted way of living.

Chapter 12

Scalp and Hair – Rooted in Nature

Walking through the hair care aisle feels like stepping into a world of promises, with every bottle claiming to transform your hair into silky strands or bouncy curls. Billboards outside show actresses with perfect, glossy waves, their hair bouncing as if it's never seen a bad day. The shelves are lined with colorful bottles, each one offering a new solution: strength, volume, shine, anti-dandruff, anti-frizz. You name it, they have it. Each claim sounds convincing, as though every bottle holds the secret to hair that's healthier, shinier, and effortlessly beautiful. Words like "infused with Moroccan argan oil," "rejuvenating silk proteins," and "botanical repair" jump out, wrapped in packaging that makes each product feel like it's exactly what our hair has been waiting for.

In this sea of choices, it's tempting to pick whatever sounds best in the moment, chasing the latest trends in hair care. But with all these options, we rarely pause to consider what our hair truly needs—or to question the long list of ingredients printed on the back of each bottle.

Behind the sleek packaging and bold claims, many products carry hidden chemicals: sulfates that create a satisfying lather but strip the hair of natural oils, silicones that add temporary gloss but build up over time, preservatives and synthetic fragrances that linger far longer than we think.

So, let's step back and rethink what our hair care routine is really giving us.

Instead of going for the next quick fix, it may be time to calm the noise, see beyond the flashy promises, and think about a more gentle approach—one that nourishes from the roots and respects the health of both our bodies and the world around us.

The Dangers of Chemical Hair Products

Once we look beyond the labels, the ingredients in many hair care products tell a different story. For all the promises of softness, shine, and strength, the list of chemicals behind these results can have effects that extend far beyond the short-term benefits.

Let's explore what's inside these bottles and how each ingredient contributes to hair care routines, the long-term health of our bodies, and the environment.

Sulfates

Sulfates, like sodium lauryl sulfate (SLS) and sodium laureth sulfate (SLES), are what make shampoos lather into that rich foam that feels like it's deeply cleansing the scalp. But while the bubbles might seem satisfying, they come at a cost. Sulfates are strong detergents that strip the scalp of its natural oils, often leaving it feeling dry and sometimes even irritated. This can trigger the scalp to produce extra oil in an effort to compensate, creating a cycle where hair feels greasier between washes, pushing us to wash more frequently. A study from *The Journal of Cosmetic Dermatology* (2022) highlights that prolonged exposure to sulfates can weaken the scalp's natural barrier, leading to flakiness and a lack of moisture balance over time.

Parabens

Parabens are preservatives used to prolong the shelf life of shampoos, conditioners, and other hair products. They prevent bacterial growth, which might sound beneficial, but parabens come with their own set of risks. Research from *The Journal of Applied Toxicology* (2023) shows that parabens can mimic estrogen in the body, potentially disrupting hormonal balance with frequent use. This means that, over time, these synthetic preservatives may interfere with natural hormone functions, impacting everything from energy levels to reproductive health. Parabens are often listed on labels as methylparaben, propylparaben, or butylparaben, so taking a quick glance at the ingredient list can help avoid these hidden additives.

Phthalates

Often found within the label of "fragrance," phthalates are used to help scents last longer, making hair products smell fresh and fragrant throughout the day. However, these chemicals don't stop at a pleasant aroma. Studies published in *The Indian Journal of Public Health* (2022) link phthalates to potential endocrine disruption, meaning they can interfere with our hormonal systems. Prolonged exposure to phthalates has been associated with reproductive health issues, especially concerning for those who use fragranced products regularly. Since phthalates are hidden under the generic term "fragrance," it's easy to miss their presence altogether, making it important to question overly perfumed products and consider the lasting effects of these invisible chemicals.

Silicones

Silicones, like dimethicone, are frequently added to conditioners and serums to give hair a smooth, shiny finish. These ingredients coat each strand, making hair feel instantly softer and less frizzy. While this effect may seem appealing, silicones do more than just add a quick gloss. Over time, they build up on the scalp and hair, creating a barrier that can clog follicles and weigh down the strands. This accumulation can hinder hair growth and leave hair feeling limp. Research from *The Journal of Dermatology and Cosmetology* (2023) emphasizes that long-term silicone buildup can even lead to scalp issues, affecting the overall health and vibrancy of the hair.

Synthetic Fragrances

Beyond phthalates, synthetic fragrances in hair products often contain VOCs (volatile organic compounds) that evaporate into the air and can impact indoor air quality. With repeated use in enclosed spaces like bathrooms, these VOCs can lead to headaches, dizziness, and respiratory issues, especially for those with sensitivities. VOCs aren't a passing concern—they linger in the air, affecting both us and those around us.

The cumulative effect of these gases, according to environmental health studies, can contribute to poor indoor air quality and may lead to more serious health issues with prolonged exposure.

Each wash, each spray, and each dye we apply in the bathroom extends far beyond our immediate surroundings. These everyday actions, which seem so contained, leave traces that reach well beyond the sink or shower.

As these chemicals travel, they affect the air we breathe, the water we drink, and the ecosystems we rely on. But when we understand the broader impact of our hair care choices, we see why these products leave an imprint that goes much further than the bathroom shelf.

The Chain Reaction on Environment

Each wash, spray, and dye we apply in the bathroom extends far beyond our immediate surroundings. These everyday actions, which seem so contained, leave traces that reach well beyond the sink or shower. The chemicals in our hair care routines travel, affecting the air we breathe, the water we drink, and the ecosystems that sustain life. Understanding the broader impact of these products helps us see how even small choices can have lasting effects on the world around us.

Aerosol hair sprays and dry shampoos, for instance, release volatile organic compounds (VOCs) into the air. While they provide convenience and quick results, their invisible emissions impact more than we realize.

In small, enclosed spaces like bathrooms, these VOCs linger long after use, affecting indoor air quality. Research from *The Environmental Health Perspectives Journal* (2023) points out that VOCs contribute to the formation of ground-level ozone, exacerbating air pollution and respiratory problems, especially in urban areas where pollution levels are already high. Each spritz, seemingly insignificant, accumulates over time, affecting not just us but the air we all share.

Hair dyes come with a hidden concern, especially those that contain ammonia and hydrogen peroxide. While the strong smell of hair dye may be recognizable, the effects of its fumes often go unnoticed. Studies from *The International Journal of Environmental Research and Public Health* (2023) show that hair salon workers, who are exposed to these chemicals regularly, face higher rates of respiratory issues. In enclosed spaces, like salons or home bathrooms, these fumes can linger, posing risks to anyone who breathes them in.What appears to be a simple refresh or color change can leave behind unseen traces that impact more than just the user.

Beyond what we breathe, the chemicals in hair products often find their way into our waterways, carried by the simple act of rinsing out shampoo, conditioner, or dye. Ingredients like silicones and certain preservatives don't break down easily and accumulate in aquatic environments. This buildup in water systems is not fixed; it travels up the food chain through a process called biological magnification. Small amounts of these substances found in fish and other marine life can accumulate to higher levels in the predators that eat them, including humans. Research from The Journal of Environmental Sciences (2023) highlights how this cycle affects biodiversity and poses risks to human health. Every time we use a product and send it down the drain, we often unknowingly contribute to this chain reaction.

The impact on aquatic life extends further. Chemicals like ammonia from hair dyes are particularly harsh on fish and aquatic plants, disrupting delicate ecosystems and reducing biodiversity. Preservatives like triclosan, common in various hair care items, can lead to antibiotic resistance in aquatic bacteria, further straining the balance of these environments. The water we rinse out isn't gone—it becomes part of a larger system that affects the health of rivers, lakes, and oceans, and everything that depends on them.

Even the way we dispose of these products matters. Tossing out leftover hair dye or empty aerosol cans can lead to chemicals leaching into the soil. Rinsing out dyes in the sink introduces pollutants into water treatment systems that may not fully filter them out. This means harmful substances can end up in fields, rivers, and habitats, impacting plants, animals, and, eventually, people.

The simple choices we make, from using products to disposing of them, have effects that extend to parts of the environment we might never see but rely on every day. With every application, every rinse, and every discard, we shape the world around us. Recognizing these impacts is the first step toward change, understanding that the effects of our routines extend far beyond ourselves.

What's often overlooked is the privilege that comes with being able to choose these products in the first place. The glossy bottles and neatly packaged solutions are often within reach only for those who can afford them, while the consequences of their use and disposal first affect those who can't. Communities living closer to polluted waterways, agricultural fields exposed to contaminated runoff, and areas with fewer resources to combat environmental degradation bear the brunt of these impacts. The very people who contribute the least to the problem often feel its effects most acutely.

Reevaluating our choices and recognizing the invisible connections that link us to others and our shared world is the first step. Each thoughtful decision becomes a responsible act, balancing privilege with the understanding that our habits can either support or burden the systems that sustain us all.

This shift in awareness opens the door to alternatives that align with both personal well-being and environmental respect—alternatives rooted in nature and tradition.

Natural Hair Care

For generations, natural ingredients have been trusted for their ability to nourish and protect the scalp and hair without the burden of harsh chemicals. These time-tested solutions have been a part of traditional care routines, offering effective results that are gentle on both the body and the environment. Embracing these natural methods can bring balance and simplicity to your hair care routine while promoting sustainable practices that benefit more than just you.

Hair Wash with Natural Ingredients

These ingredients often provide additional benefits such as moisturizing the scalp, enhancing hair strength, and even promoting hair growth. By incorporating natural elements into your hair washing routine, you engage in a practice that nourishes and revitalizes your hair without compromising on your health or the environment.

Shikakai and Reetha (Soapnut) Cleansing

Shikakai and reetha have long been staples in traditional Ayurvedic hair care. Shikakai, often referred to as "fruit for the hair," is a natural cleanser that removes dirt and excess oil without stripping away the scalp's essential moisture. Its mild acidic nature helps maintain the scalp's natural pH, reducing dandruff and promoting healthy hair growth. Reetha, on the other hand, is rich in saponins that produce a gentle lather, offering a satisfying cleanse without the synthetic foaming agents found in modern shampoos.

To use, soak reetha pods overnight, boil them in water until the liquid thickens, and strain. Mix this infusion with shikakai powder or use it on its own as a hair cleanser. The result is clean, soft, and nourished hair with enhanced manageability and shine. Over time, this natural routine can help reduce hair fall and improve scalp health.

Urad Dal Powder Cleaner

Urad dal (black gram) may not be the first ingredient that comes to mind for hair care, but its high protein and vitamin content make it a powerful cleanser and conditioner. When ground into a fine powder and mixed with water or yogurt, urad dal creates a natural hair pack that gently removes impurities while strengthening hair strands. This remedy is especially beneficial for dry or damaged hair, as it provides deep nourishment and helps restore natural elasticity and shine.

Multani Mitti Paste for Cleansing

Multani mitti, or Fuller's earth, is known for its ability to absorb excess oil and cleanse deeply, making it an excellent choice for oily or greasy hair. Its mineral-rich composition not only detoxifies the scalp but also helps unclog hair follicles, promoting healthier hair growth. To prepare, mix multani mitti with water or rose water into a smooth paste and apply it to your scalp and hair. Leave it on for 10-15 minutes before rinsing with lukewarm water. This treatment is particularly helpful for those dealing with an oily scalp or product buildup.

Black Soil for Hair Cleansing

Black soil, an age-old remedy, has been traditionally used in rural communities to cleanse and strengthen hair. Rich in minerals and completely natural, it gently exfoliates the scalp, removes impurities, and enhances circulation, which can improve hair growth. To use, mix clean, sifted black soil with water to create a paste, apply it to the scalp, and massage gently before rinsing thoroughly. This method is not only effective but also deeply rooted in sustainable living practices, showcasing how the earth itself provides solutions for self-care.

Hair Care

Natural hair care focuses on creating a balanced routine that works harmoniously with your scalp and hair's natural needs. Just like skin, hair thrives when treated with care, and natural ingredients offer a way to restore and maintain that balance. Applying oil to the scalp provides essential nourishment, promoting scalp health, which in turn supports strong and healthy hair follicles.

Choose an oil that suits you—whether it's mustard, sesame, coconut, amla, or even ghee—and massage it into your scalp twice a week for optimal results. Beyond these options, the following oils are worth considering to enhance your hair care routine and deserve a spot on your shelf.

Jojoba Oil

Jojoba oil is known for its unique ability to mimic the natural oils produced by the scalp. This makes it an ideal moisturizer that hydrates without clogging pores or weighing down the hair. Its lightweight texture penetrates deeply, balancing sebum production and leaving the scalp refreshed. According to *The Indian Journal of Dermatology* (2022), jojoba oil is particularly helpful for those with oily scalps, as it provides moisture without contributing to buildup. A few drops massaged into the scalp can keep hair nourished and healthy.

Argan Oil

Often called "liquid gold," argan oil is rich in essential fatty acids and vitamin E. This oil is cherished for its ability to restore shine and strengthen dry or damaged hair. Used as a leave-in treatment, argan oil hydrates deeply, protecting hair from environmental stressors and reducing frizz. Its nutrient-rich profile makes it perfect for revitalizing hair that needs a bit of extra care, whether from heat styling or daily exposure to the sun and pollutants.

Aloe Vera

Aloe vera is celebrated for its cooling and soothing properties, making it a natural remedy for an itchy or irritated scalp. Applied directly, aloe vera gel reduces inflammation and provides a dose of hydration, perfect for sensitive scalps that react to harsh chemicals. Many households keep an aloe vera plant, finding comfort in its simple, natural relief. Applying fresh aloe gel or store-bought aloe vera without additives can calm the scalp and keep it moisturized, helping maintain a healthy base for strong hair.

Apple Cider Vinegar Rinse

An apple cider vinegar rinse is a straightforward way to remove residue and restore the scalp's natural pH balance. This rinse not only keeps hair shiny but helps maintain scalp health without disrupting its natural oils. To use, dilute apple cider vinegar with water and apply it as a final rinse after shampooing. The mild acidity helps clarify the scalp and hair, leaving a natural shine that feels clean and light. This simple step can be a refreshing alternative to store-bought clarifying products, offering results without synthetic additives.

Each of these natural methods offers a way to bring balance and care into your hair care routine, but incorporating them into daily life can take some adjustment. Switching from synthetic products to natural alternatives doesn't happen overnight, and it's important to be patient with yourself as your hair and scalp adapt. The transition is worth it, helping your hair achieve a natural shine and health that comes without the hidden trade-offs of chemical-based products.

Implementation of Natural Products

Transitioning to natural hair care can feel different, especially if you've spent years using commercial shampoos, conditioners, and styling products. The scalp and hair might respond in unexpected ways at first, but with a little patience and some practical guidance, this shift can be both smooth and rewarding. Here are some tips to help you make the most of your natural hair care journey.

Gradual Integration

Start slow. If you're used to conventional shampoos and conditioners, introducing natural products gradually is key. Begin by alternating between your regular shampoo and a natural one, such as a mild shikakai or reetha-based cleanser. This approach helps your scalp adjust without sudden changes that might leave your hair feeling greasy or dry. Over time, as your scalp releases the buildup from synthetic ingredients, you'll notice a more natural balance in oil production and overall texture. Think of this phase as a gentle reset, allowing your hair to find its true state without the interference of harsh chemicals.

Understanding the Adjustment Period

It's normal for your scalp to go through an adjustment period when you first switch to natural products. You might notice your hair feeling oilier or even drier than usual during the first couple of weeks. This is simply your scalp recalibrating as it sheds the remnants of silicones and sulfates that previously stripped it of its natural oils. Research from *The Journal of Clinical Dermatology* (2023) notes that within a few weeks, most people's scalps adapt, and the oil production finds its natural rhythm. Know that this temporary phase can be a challenge but knowing that it leads to healthier hair will help you stay committed.

Application Techniques for Different Hair Types

Everyone's hair is different, and understanding how to use natural products to suit your specific hair type makes all the difference.

- **Curly or Dry Hair**:Curly hair needs moisture, and jojoba oil is great for that. After washing your hair, just apply a few drops of jojoba oil to damp hair, especially on the ends where dryness often appears. Jojoba oil's lightweight properties allow it to hydrate deeply without making curls heavy, enhancing their natural shape and reducing frizz. In absence of Jojoba oil any other oil can be used.
- **Straight or Fine Hair**: If your hair is straight or fine, use argan oil sparingly as a leave-in conditioner. Just a couple of drops smoothed onto the hair, especially on the ends, can add a healthy shine and moisture without making the hair look greasy or flat. This method helps maintain the volume and softness that straight and fine hair needs.
- **Sensitive Scalps**: For those with sensitive scalps prone to irritation, aloe vera gel can be a soothing savior. Apply a thin layer directly to the scalp, massaging it in gently. Let it sit for around 15 minutes before rinsing it out with lukewarm water. This simple step can calm inflammation, reduce itchiness, and leave the scalp feeling refreshed and balanced.

Regular Apple Cider Vinegar Rinses

Incorporating an apple cider vinegar rinse once a week can work wonders for maintaining a balanced scalp and removing product buildup naturally. Mix one part apple cider vinegar with three parts water, pour it over your scalp after shampooing, and let it sit for a few minutes before rinsing thoroughly. This helps cleanse without the harshness of clarifying shampoos that strip the hair, leaving it smoother and more manageable.

These techniques are simple but powerful ways to care for your hair while staying mindful of the products you use. Embracing natural care is an invitation to move beyond the quick fixes and embrace a more thoughtful, balanced approach to your well-being.

When we rethink our hair care routines, we're making a choice that's deeper than what meets the eye. We're choosing to align with practices that honor not only our body but the environment that sustains us. Each step, from a nourishing oil massage to a gentle rinse, speaks to a commitment to care that is rooted in simplicity and intention. It's a shift that values long-term health over temporary results and mindful action over convenience.

This approach echoes the care taken by generations before us, where natural remedies were chosen not out of trend but out of trust in what was known to nurture and protect. In today's fast-paced world, reconnecting with these practices is a way to slow down and prioritize what truly supports us, reminding ourselves that small, deliberate choices can lead to meaningful change.

As you move forward, think of each natural practice not as a replacement, but as an act of respect—for your hair, your health, and the wider world that each choice touches.

These habits carry more than personal benefit; they are a nod to traditions that valued harmony and sustainability. In choosing them, you're not only caring for yourself but contributing to a greater cycle of balance and mindfulness that extends beyond you.

True care is found in the choices we make every day, the moments where simplicity meets intention, and where we find balance in nurturing both ourselves and the world we call home.

Chapter 13

Cooking and Eating – The Chemical Diet

Do you remember your favorite meal growing up?

The one that filled the house with that familiar smell and brought everyone to the table. Maybe it was your grandmother's curry simmering in her old kadhai, or fresh chapatis puffing up over the flame. The kitchen was alive, filled with the scent of warm spices and the gentle clatter of pots and pans. Every meal felt like it was made with care, and every ingredient had a place.

Now, think about your kitchen today. The shiny non-stick pans, the prepackaged sauces that promise flavor without effort, the rows of bright bottles lined up on the counter. From the preservatives in bread to the chemicals coating your non-stick pan, our kitchens hold more than just ingredients for a meal—they tell a story of convenience, chemicals, and quiet compromises.

You reach for a familiar pan, light and easy to handle, and gather ingredients. There's a moment when your eyes drift to the labels on jars and packets, words that are hard to pronounce, even harder to understand. When did cooking, once so simple and rooted in tradition, take on this extra layer? Additives in our food, coatings on our pans, shortcuts that seemed so helpful but might have hidden costs.

What slipped into our kitchens over time? What do all these extras mean for our health? Maybe it's time to take a closer look at what we're really bringing to our tables and what these choices mean for us—beyond the surface.

Chemicals in the Kitchen

You place the pan on the stove, add a little oil, and hear that satisfying sizzle as it heats up. Non-stick pans make cooking feel easy. They save time, reduce the need for oil, and make cleanup a breeze. But beneath that convenience lies a story we rarely see: a coating that can release invisible fumes, a material that might be safer at first but has consequences that stick around far longer than we realize.

Non-stick pans, often coated with polytetrafluoroethylene (PTFE), commonly known as Teflon, have transformed cooking. PTFE provides that smooth, non-stick surface, preventing food from sticking even with little oil. However, when these pans are overheated—going above 260°C (500°F)—they begin to release fumes that can impact the air we breathe. Studies in *Environmental Science & Technology* (2023) show that PTFE fumes, once inhaled, can cause "polymer fume fever," leading to flu-like symptoms. In a kitchen with limited ventilation, these fumes can build up, posing risks to respiratory health, especially for those with conditions like asthma.

Beyond our kitchens, there's an environmental footprint that non-stick pans carry. PTFE coatings, for instance, don't decompose easily. Once discarded, they end up in landfills, where they can persist for decades, potentially leaching chemicals into surrounding soil and water. Each pan might not seem significant, but imagine the accumulation over time, with countless non-stick pans discarded year after year.

Then there's aluminum cookware. Lightweight, durable, and affordable, aluminum pans and pots have been a kitchen staple for decades. They heat evenly and make cooking feel effortless. However, cooking acidic foods like tomatoes or tamarind in aluminum can cause tiny amounts of the metal to seep into the food. Research from *The Journal of Food Safety* (2022) suggests that regular exposure to aluminum, even in small amounts, can build up in the body, potentially affecting neurological health over the long term.

The journey of aluminum doesn't begin in our kitchens—it starts in mines, often deep within forests, where the extraction process disrupts entire ecosystems. Aluminum production demands large amounts of energy, contributing to greenhouse gas emissions and habitat loss. The mining process leaves scars on the landscape, while the disposal of aluminum products adds yet another layer of waste to landfills. Each step, from extraction to disposal, carries a cost that goes unnoticed in the shiny, practical surface of our cookware.

These are the hidden details that don't make it to the product labels, details that get buried beneath layers of convenience and practicality. When we use these products daily, it's easy to overlook what they leave behind—for us, for our homes, and for the world outside our kitchens. Understanding these hidden layers helps us see beyond the ease and efficiency, encouraging us to think about what we truly want to bring into our kitchens and our lives.

Food Additives

As we look closer at what's in our kitchens, our gaze shifts from the cookware to the food itself, especially the processed foods that have become everyday staples. Packaged foods fill the shelves of every kirana store, from instant noodles like Maggi and Yippee to the bright snack packets promising flavor in every bite. Each item feels like a familiar friend on the shelf, offering convenience and comfort, a quick fix for when time runs short or hunger strikes. But that rich taste, the color that catches your eye, and the long shelf life of these snacks don't come naturally. Behind the crisp flavors and vibrant packaging are carefully added chemicals, extending freshness, enhancing flavor, and ensuring that satisfying crunch. While these additives make life easier, they bring hidden costs that go beyond what we taste or see.

Take the preservatives that keep our favorite snacks from spoiling too soon. In popular treats and ready-to-eat meals, chemicals like butylated hydroxyanisole (BHA) and butylated hydroxytoluene (BHT) are used to prevent oils from going stale. Their purpose is straightforward—no one wants a biscuit that tastes old or a chip that's lost its crispness. Yet behind this practicality lies a deeper layer. According to *The International Journal of Toxicology* (2023), BHA has been identified as a potential human carcinogen, with links to hormone disruption when consumed regularly over time. So, while a single snack may seem harmless, regularly eating foods with these additives leads to a slow buildup in our bodies, creating risks that may not be visible but are there nonetheless.

Beyond our personal health, there's the broader environmental impact of these synthetic preservatives. BHA and BHT are derived from petrochemicals and involve energy-intensive production processes that release greenhouse gases and pollutants into the atmosphere. The manufacturing of these additives leaves behind more than flavor; it contributes to climate change and air pollution, effects that often go unnoticed but touch every breath we take. Each time we reach for a packet of chips or instant noodles, we indirectly support this cycle, where the comfort of a quick snack is linked to environmental consequences far beyond the snack itself.

Then there's monosodium glutamate (MSG), a flavor enhancer found in everything from instant soups to noodle packets. Known for its savory kick, MSG has become a staple in processed foods, delivering that irresistible umami taste in everything from packaged masalas to instant curry mixes. But while it certainly intensifies flavor, MSG has been associated with health concerns like headaches, bloating, and digestive discomfort, especially with frequent consumption. Studies from *The Indian Journal of Nutrition and Dietetics* (2023) reveal that MSG may even worsen certain health conditions, raising important questions about its presence in foods that have become staples in our homes.

The impact of producing flavor enhancers like MSG extends beyond personal health, touching on the environment. To meet the high demand for these additives, agriculture often relies on heavy applications of chemical fertilizers and pesticides, creating strains on soil health and contaminating water sources. These chemicals leach into rivers and lakes, harming aquatic life and disrupting the delicate ecosystems that support biodiversity. Over time, soil degradation and polluted waters lead to reduced crop yields and a decline in wildlife, a loss that affects not only the environment but the entire cycle of food production.

Each time we pick up a product containing these additives, we engage in a cycle that reaches from the fields to our tables. From the fertilizers used to grow the crops to the factories where these synthetic compounds are made, our choices affect more than what's on our plates.

Understanding the layers of production and the journey these foods take, helps us gain a new awareness of what we're really choosing—and what we're supporting—each time we go for convenience over simplicity.

Our kitchens, which used to be filled with fresh ingredients and careful preparation, now contain items with invisible effects that go well beyond just taste and convenience. So, each meal becomes a chance to rethink what we're bringing into our bodies and how these choices impact the world around us.

Seasonal Fruit Consumption and Agricultural Practices

When was the last time you strolled through a market, weaving through rows of colorful produce stacked high? The sight is tempting, familiar, and so abundant that we rarely pause to reflect. There was a time when these fruits appeared only once a year, their arrival eagerly anticipated and celebrated. I am not dwelling deep into it here as this subject is as long as a book in itself.

But, for your understanding, let me cite a few examples - Mangoes and Melons are summer fruits, Guavas are winter special—while staples like bananas, sweet lime, and papayas are available year-round.

Today, we fill our baskets without a second thought, rarely stopping to ask how or why this endless variety is always within reach.This year-round abundance comes at a hidden cost.

To keep up with year-round demand, industrial agriculture leans heavily on synthetic fertilizers and pesticides, working overtime to produce crops that were once seasonal. These practices, while convenient, have far-reaching effects that impact everything from soil health to the water we drink.

Soil, which naturally flourishes with seasonal crop rotations and organic nutrients, starts to suffer when fed a steady diet of chemical fertilizers. Over time, these additives deplete the soil, stripping away essential nutrients and breaking down its natural structure. Reports from *The Indian Journal of Environmental Studies* (2023) highlight how soils treated heavily with synthetic fertilizers become more compact and lose their ability to retain water, making it harder to sustain crops season after season. Instead of rejuvenating itself, the soil becomes dependent on more chemicals, starting a cycle that's tough to break and leading to erosion and degradation that can last for decades.

The reach of these chemicals doesn't stop at the soil.

When pesticides and fertilizers are applied to fields, they often end up in nearby water sources through runoff, especially after rain. This means that rivers, lakes, and even groundwater start to carry traces of these chemicals. Contaminated water affects more than just the fields it flows through; it impacts entire communities. The *World Health Organization* has expressed growing concern over pesticide residues in drinking water, warning of long-term health risks, particularly in agricultural regions where clean water is already a limited resource. For families, farmers, and livestock that depend on these water sources, the presence of chemicals adds an unseen layer of risk.

Then, there's the question of biodiversity. Every field treated with pesticides loses more than just pests—it loses the natural pollinators that help crops grow and keep ecosystems balanced. Bees, butterflies, and other pollinators that support a wide range of plants and flowers struggle in areas filled with chemicals. As they disappear, food crops suffer, leading to reduced yields and a less resilient food system. The impact doesn't stop with pollinators; other species that once thrived in these habitats face disruption as farmland expands and chemicals alter the land, causing a decline in native plants and animals essential to local ecosystems.

So, as we fill our baskets with the fruits of every season, it's worth considering the true cost of this abundance. Out-of-season produce may bring a momentary pleasure, but often at the expense of our soil, water, and biodiversity. Supporting seasonal produce helps us respect the natural cycles that keep our food systems healthy and protect our ecosystems.

Each meal is a chance to connect with nature's rhythms, enjoy food at its best, and make choices that nurture both our bodies and the environment. Every choice, from the pan we use to the vegetables we chop, reflects values that shape our health, our communities, and the land we rely on.

So, as we consider each choice we make in the kitchen, there's a growing sense that simple, thoughtful selections bring a deeper kind of nourishment. Our elders knew this, leaning toward items that were as lasting as they were useful. A sturdy kadhai, a tempered glass jar, or that treasured stainless steel tiffin box—these were items chosen not for convenience alone but for how they quietly supported health and care over time. They weren't merely practical; they connected the act of cooking to a larger, enduring respect for the food, the people, and the world that sustained us.

Wholesome Alternatives

In many ways, the cookware we choose becomes part of the flavor and care in our meals. Beyond convenience, cookware made of enduring materials like cast iron, stainless steel, and glass brings safety and quality into the kitchen, free of the risks found in synthetic coatings or disposable utensils. As we reimagine what we place in our kitchens, these timeless materials offer both peace of mind and a connection to natural, uncomplicated ways of preparing food.

Cast Iron

Cast iron has long held a special place in traditional cooking. Known for its strength and even heating, a cast iron pan, once seasoned, becomes naturally non-stick without the need for synthetic layers. Studies in the *Journal of Sustainable Home Practices* (2023) highlight how, unlike Teflon, cast iron doesn't leach chemicals into food and can last generations. Beyond its practical appeal, cast iron brings a certain richness to cooking that only grows with each meal, making it a staple for those who value both durability and the deep, flavorful results it creates.

Glass and Stainless Steel

Glass and stainless steel, too, are invaluable for any kitchen aiming for balance between safety and versatility. Unlike reactive metals, glass cookware is perfect for acidic dishes—think tamarind-based curries or simmered tomatoes—without changing flavor or releasing unwanted elements. Stainless steel, meanwhile, offers durability and ease, withstanding high temperatures while remaining easy to maintain. Both materials support a kind of cooking that doesn't involve chemicals or coating, letting us focus on the food itself and how it nourishes.

Choosing Organic Foods

The ingredients we choose have an impact that extends far past the plate. Opting for organic produce helps reduce our exposure to pesticides while also supporting farming practices that enrich rather than deplete the soil. Organic foods are grown without synthetic chemicals, offering nutrients and flavors that reflect the earth they come from, untouched by harmful additives. According to findings from the *Indian Council of Agricultural Research (ICAR)*, organic farming enhances biodiversity, protects water sources, and nurtures a more balanced ecosystem that benefits everyone along the food chain.

Beginning with a few basics—like greens, seasonal fruits, or grains—can ease the shift to organic. These choices connect us with foods grown with care, a way of eating that supports farmers who prioritize sustainability and strengthens the natural cycles that keep our food systems resilient.

Practical Tips for Sustainable Living

There's beauty in making small, intentional changes that bring both health and joy to our kitchens.

Farmers' Markets

Visiting farmers' markets allows us to explore fresh, seasonal foods while supporting the farmers who grow them. There's a richness in seeing the plump tomatoes, leafy greens, and fragrant herbs displayed by the very people who cultivated them. Shopping directly from local farmers gives us food that's fresher, often more flavorful, and grown in alignment with natural cycles. Each item, from bright coriander bunches to sweet carrots, brings the flavor of the season, reminding us of the unique tastes that local markets offer. This way we will also help in uplifting them economically and they will think about growing more once they start earning directly from consumers (which is you and I).

Home Gardens

A small home garden—whether a few pots of tulsi, fresh green chilies, or a curry leaf plant—adds freshness to meals while reducing the need for store-bought items. Each handful of mint or fresh tomato plucked from a your pot or your backyard plant offers the satisfaction of growing something directly, of knowing exactly where it came from and the care that went into it. Even the smallest harvest brings joy and adds flavor, reminding us of the simple pleasure in nurturing ingredients from seed to plate.

Reusable Kitchen Solutions

Replacing single-use items with durable, reusable alternatives can transform our kitchens into spaces of intentional care. Swapping plastic wraps for beeswax covers, single-use tissue and towels for cloth alternatives, and disposable bags for stainless steel containers are easy ways to cut down on waste. Each item becomes a small investment in sustainability, reducing our reliance on disposables and aligning our daily habits with a gentler impact on the planet.

The scent of spices, the feel of warm steam rising from a simmering pot, the sound of vegetables sizzling on the stovetop—our kitchens hold so much more than ingredients. They hold our memories, our family traditions, and the quiet routines that ground us. Each meal is a reminder of all the small choices we make, decisions that impact the world in ways we may never fully see but somehow feel. It's these choices—of ingredients, of tools, of mindful practices—that form the soul of our kitchens, shaping a space that nurtures us and those we care for.

As we move through our days, rushing or taking our time, reaching for familiar items or exploring new ones, there's a sense that our kitchens can be places of deep connection. Each spoonful, each stir, is a chance to honor the simplicity our elders cherished—a way of cooking that didn't need additives, shortcuts, or throwaway items. They knew, perhaps without saying, that a well-loved kadhai, a wooden spatula, or a handful of fresh herbs carried meaning beyond its purpose. These choices reflected respect: respect for the food itself, for those who grew it, and for the land that made it possible.

So, as we cook each meal, we have an opportunity to continue this respect. We can choose tools that don't harm our health or the planet, select ingredients that nourish fully, and adopt habits that don't rely on convenience alone. With each mindful step, our kitchens become places of warmth, resilience, and care. They become spaces where health and tradition come together naturally, a space where the simple act of cooking transforms into a gesture of kindness—for our bodies, our communities, and the earth.

In choosing thoughtfully, we're reminded that each meal is a connection to something larger, a way to live gently within the world's rhythms, sharing in its abundance without taking more than we need. This approach brings us closer to what matters, creating a kitchen and life filled with intention, balance, and gratitude. And each day, as we stir, chop, and share these meals, we're part of a story much older than us, a story of simplicity and care that we can continue, honoring all that came before and all that lies ahead.

Section 3

Advocating for a Better Tomorrow

Chapter 14

Coexisting with Nature – The Benefits of Rooted Living

Breathe in deeply for a moment. Let me ask you something—

When was the last time you touched the soil? Not while rushing through chores or brushing past it on your way somewhere, but with purpose—letting it crumble between your fingers, cool and grounding. When was the last time you breathed in the rich scent of the earth after the first rain, that unmistakable petrichor that seems to awaken something deep within? Or paused to hear the rustling of leaves, the quiet rhythm of nature's whispers cutting through the hum of the everyday? These simple acts, once familiar and constant, now feel rare—moments we've traded for hurried routines and endless screens.

In the last chapter, we explored how nature's cycles inspire ways of living that regenerate rather than deplete. These ideas aren't abstract; they start with us—with the choices we make in our homes, kitchens, and communities. They remind us that the systems we build and the habits we form can either connect us to the natural world or pull us further away from it. Somewhere along the way, though, we've drifted. Concrete has replaced open spaces, and the quiet hum of the earth has been drowned out by the noise of busy lives.

Yet, the earth hasn't forgotten us. Its rhythm continues in the rise and fall of seasons, in the way a monsoon transforms the soil, and in the quiet persistence of roots breaking through cracks in the pavement.

So, what would it mean to pause, to notice, and to realign with these cycles—not as an obligation, but as a way of finding balance?

Perhaps the first step isn't a grand gesture, but a simple, thoughtful choice—a chance to reconnect with the earth beneath our feet and rediscover what we've always belonged to.

Rediscovering the benefits of Rooted Living

The cycles of nature continue, steady and unchanging, even as we move further away from them. The irony of the present it that this was not too long ago but, just a few decades ago – and we all know it. So, realigning back with these rhythms doesn't require a complete transformation; it's more like returning to something familiar and grounding. This is what rooted living means—a way of being that mirrors the simplicity and interconnectedness of the natural world. It's waking up with the first light of dawn, not the sharp ring of an alarm, and savoring the sweetness of a mango in the height of summer, rather than an imported version that's lost its flavor. It's choosing the fresh air of an early evening walk over the glow of a screen or the hum of artificial lights. These small changes bring a sense of balance and connection, making life feel more in tune with the world around us.

Think of a family who started making small shifts in how they lived. They stopped buying fruits and vegetables grown with chemicals and planted their own instead, using water collected from the rain. Their roof is lined with solar panels, and they cook meals with fresh ingredients grown just steps from their kitchen. Over time, they noticed they felt healthier, spent less money, and felt closer to the earth. These changes didn't happen all at once, but each small step made their lives feel more whole.

This isn't something only families are doing. In some neighborhoods, composting has become a way to bring people together. Families save their vegetable peels, tea leaves, and other scraps to add to a shared composting pile. Over time, those scraps turn into rich soil that helps grow flowers, fruits, and vegetables in local gardens. The benefits are more than practical—people meet, share ideas, and form connections that make the neighborhood stronger and more united!

There are also businesses learning from nature's cycles. One makes plates from leaves—strong, reusable, and able to return to the soil without leaving any waste. Another turns husks and stems from crops into packaging, showing that even the leftovers of farming can have a new use. These ideas do more than solve problems—they show how working with nature can lead to creative and lasting solutions.

This way of living also changes how we feel. Sitting in the sunlight helps us sleep better, strengthens our immunity, and lifts our mood. Breathing clean air, far from the noise and pollution of busy streets, refreshes the body and clears the mind. Eating fruits and vegetables when they're in season gives us the nutrition our bodies naturally need.

Research shows how much these connections actually help us: a study in *The Journal of Environmental Psychology* (2023) found that spending even a short time in a green space can lower stress, improve focus, and spark creativity. That's why walking under shady trees or sitting by a quiet river leaves us feeling calm and clear-headed. These simple moments help us feel grounded in a way that nothing else can.

Rooted living isn't a step backward. It's a way to move forward by finding simple, thoughtful ways to live. It helps us reconnect with what keeps us healthy and steady.

The Synergy Between Personal and Planetary Well-Being

The way we choose to live shapes our health, happiness, and the world we share. Our actions extend outward, affecting ecosystems, the air we breathe, and the water we rely on. Rooted living creates a sense of harmony for ourselves and the earth beneath us. The connection is simple: what sustains us also sustains the planet, and what harms the planet eventually harms us.

Take the air around us. When we switch to natural cleaning products, for instance, we avoid harsh chemicals in our homes while reducing the release of volatile organic compounds (VOCs) that pollute the air outside. These small changes, multiplied across communities, result in cleaner air for everyone, especially in cities where pollution is already a challenge. The choices we make indoors extend far beyond the walls of our homes.

Or think of the fabrics we wear. Choosing organic cotton over synthetic materials goes beyond comfort. It protects the soil where these crops grow. Synthetic fabrics depend on chemical-heavy farming and processing, depleting soil nutrients and contaminating water tables. Organic farming preserves the land, keeping it fertile and healthy for future crops. Each choice influences more than what we wear—it shapes the land we depend on.

The connection between rooted living and biodiversity runs even deeper.

Supporting organic farming provides cleaner food while creating habitats for pollinators like bees and butterflies. These creatures are vital to the food we eat, pollinating fruits and vegetables. Their survival ensures the survival of the plants that sustain us, linking every meal to their essential work.

Even simple practices, like composting kitchen scraps, contribute meaningfully. A compost bin at home turns leftovers into rich, fertile soil. This soil nourishes plants, reducing the need for chemical fertilizers. Over time, composting keeps the soil alive, supporting crops for generations. Healthier soil leads to better food security, ensuring that future harvests are abundant and nutritious.

These changes are part of the small decisions we make every day: how we cook, how we store food, how we treat what's left behind. When we align these habits with nature's flow, we create a system of care that benefits everyone. The earth supports us, and in turn, we support it, forming a connection that sustains both life and well-being.

Long Term benefits of Rooted Living

As you've read in the chapters so far, even small choices can have a significant impact on the future.

Each time you repurpose, compost, or grow something of your own, you're contributing to something larger than yourself—a world that can sustain itself for generations to come. The way we live today has a direct impact on the world we pass on, shaping it into a place that either thrives or struggles under the weight of our habits. Rooted living gives us a chance to leave behind more than just footprints. It's a way of planting seeds—both literal and metaphorical—for a healthier, more resilient future.

Take something as simple as reusing water. The water leftover from rinsing grains or vegetables can nourish your plants instead of being poured down the drain. This small habit reduces waste, saves resources, and helps the greenery around you flourish. Imagine a balcony garden of fresh mint, tulsi, and coriander, grown with care and watered from your kitchen.

These plants don't only provide food; they also save you the last-minute scramble to dash downstairs for tulsi or dhaniya when your mom suddenly asks. Having them right on your balcony feels like a small victory, a simple convenience woven into daily life. Beyond that, they bring a quiet sense of calm, connecting you to the rhythm of growing and nurturing something with care. Over time, tending to them becomes part of your routine—a gentle reminder that even the smallest spaces can play a role in the larger cycle of renewal.

Growing food offers more than self-sufficiency; it reconnects us with the satisfaction of creating something with our hands. A pot of fresh tomatoes or chillies growing on your balcony is more than a source of food—it's a daily reminder of the effort and care that goes into nurturing life. Watching a seed sprout and grow, its leaves unfurling little by little, until it becomes part of a meal shared with loved ones, brings a grounding sense of accomplishment.

These small actions show that even the tiniest spaces can make a difference when approached with intention.

Rooted living also reminds us to cherish what we already have. A chipped mug doesn't need to end up in the trash—it can hold pens or house a small succulent, bringing life and purpose to something forgotten. An old saree, its fabric softened by years of use, can be repurposed into reusable shopping bags or gentle cleaning cloths. Acts like these go beyond practicality; they bring quiet satisfaction, a sense of purpose in knowing nothing is wasted. Repairing a wobbly chair or patching a favorite bag connects us to the story of these objects, honoring the resourcefulness of those who came before us.

There's also something deeply rewarding in choosing to support local farmers or artisans. Imagine picking up a basket of fruits and vegetables from a neighborhood market—their colors vibrant, their scents fresh, and their textures full of life. These aren't items that sat for days in cold storage or ripened artificially during transport. They've been nurtured close to home, by people who understand the rhythms of the land. Each item tells a story of soil, sun, and care, making every bite more meaningful. Choosing these over packaged alternatives strengthens both your meals and the bonds between communities and the land they depend on.

These mindful actions extend outward, making a measurable impact far beyond your home. Research from The Indian Council of Environmental Research (2023) shows that households adopting rooted living practices can reduce waste by 30% and significantly lower their carbon footprint. This isn't achieved through grand gestures—it's the cumulative effect of small, consistent choices.

The benefits of rooted living go beyond the physical. Growing herbs on your balcony, knowing the backstory of the food on your plate, or mending a cherished item brings a sense of connection in a fast-paced, disposable world. These acts help ground us in what truly matters—relationships, mindfulness, and living with intention. They shift the focus away from convenience and toward care, enriching not only our daily lives but also the environment we rely on.

As these habits become part of who we are, they deepen our respect for the resources that sustain us. They remind us to care for the rivers that quench our thirst, the soil that nourishes our food, and the air that fills our lungs. This respect shapes more than our present; it builds a legacy for those who come after us—a world capable of sustaining life because of the thoughtful actions of those who came before.

Balanced Living

Now, living in harmony with nature is not a task or a checklist; it is a quiet rediscovery of what it means to be part of something larger. It's a way of seeing the world that honors the connections between our actions and the lives they touch—both near and far.

Every choice we make, no matter how small, impacts our surroundings and shapes the way we see ourselves within them.

Take a moment to reflect on your day. Think of the water you used, the food you ate, the air you breathed.

Each of these is a gift from the earth, a reminder of the cycles that sustain us. When we align with these rhythms, life begins to feel less rushed, less fragmented. Cooking with fresh, seasonal ingredients, tending to a small garden, or walking through a park as sunlight filters through the trees—these aren't things that demand us to go out of our way, but they carry the weight of care and intention. They remind us that life's richness lies not in excess but in the connections we nurture.

Rooted living is not a return to the past; it's an embrace of what's timeless. It is the joy of creating something meaningful with your hands, whether that's mending a piece of clothing or growing herbs in a pot on your balcony. **It's the satisfaction of knowing that the choices you make today will leave the soil richer, the water cleaner, and the air fresher for those who come after you.**

This way of living is as much about love as it is about responsibility—a love for the world that sustains us and for the people and places that make it home.

When we shift our perspective, we begin to see abundance where before there seemed to be scarcity. An old jar becomes a container for grains, a torn saree transforms into sturdy shopping bags, and kitchen scraps turn into fertile compost.

These small acts of preservation are more than practical; they are affirmations of our ability to care deeply for what we have and to find value in what might otherwise be discarded.

And in these moments of care, something amazing begins to unfold. We find ourselves reconnecting—not only with the earth but with each other! Sharing a home-cooked meal with neighbors, exchanging seeds with friends, or simply talking about how to live more thoughtfully creates bonds that go beyond words. These connections remind us that we're not alone in this journey. Together, we can build a world where care flows between people, communities, and the environment, creating a cycle that sustains everyone.

This is not a call to do everything or to strive for perfection. It is an invitation to begin—to take one step toward a life that feels grounded and intentional. Start with what feels natural: reuse what you can, grow what's possible, and give back in ways that feel meaningful to you. Each choice, no matter how small, becomes part of a larger story—a story of renewal, respect, and resilience.

Rooted living is a reminder that we belong to the earth as much as it belongs to us. It is a way of life that honors the quiet rhythms of nature and invites us to move with them rather than against them. In choosing this path, we create a life that feels whole, not because it is perfect, but because it is connected—to the land, to the people around us, and to the generations yet to come.

This is the legacy we can leave: a world shaped by care, where every action speaks of balance and every choice carries the hope of something better.

Chapter 15

Advocating for Change

At some point, we stopped seeing the land beneath us as a partner and started treating it as something to take from. We paved over fields, boxed ourselves into concrete homes, and traded sunlight for fluorescent lights. The streams that once bubbled in the background of childhood memories became polluted channels, the sturdy clay pots our grandmothers watered plants with were replaced by plastics that crack and fade. Trees that stood tall through changing seasons became shadows of themselves, felled to make way for roads and buildings. Yet, through it all, the earth has quietly continued to provide—its cycles ensuring food, water, and air without fail.

But what happens when this balance tips?

When the soil, weakened by chemicals, no longer nourishes crops? When the rivers that once quenched our thirst turn undrinkable, carrying pollutants instead of life? When the air we breathe, thick with smoke and toxins, suffocates instead of refreshes? These constants—our food, our health, our stories—are at risk. And the question now is not simply what the earth can give us, but what it needs from us in return.

Now that we're at the final chapter, let's shift our attention back to these quiet supporters of life.It's time to see them for what they truly are:

the foundation of everything we depend on. This is not an individual effort, but a collective shift—a movement toward reclaiming harmony with the cycles that sustain us.

The time to act is now, with small, thoughtful steps that create a world where balance is restored and where we give back as much as we take.

Regulatory Challenges

As we pause to reflect on this balance, it's impossible to ignore the invisible threats that tip the scales. Imagine a quiet village by the river, where generations have drawn from its waters for drinking, cooking, and farming. Today, that same river flows murky, its surface carrying traces of industrial waste, chemicals leaching from distant factories, and residues from fields saturated with pesticides. The water that once sustained life now carries danger, its contamination seeping into the soil, the crops, and the bodies of those who unknowingly consume it.

This issue isn't as distant or remote as you'd think. It's the food on our plates, the water in our glasses, and the air we breathe every day. It's in the non-stick pans in our kitchens and the water-resistant clothes in our cupboards. These silent invaders, often called "forever chemicals," have become part of our lives without us realizing the long-term costs. Designed to resist heat, water, and grease, these substances linger in the environment indefinitely, accumulating in the soil, water, and even within us.

A report published in 2023 by the Indian Environmental Health Association highlighted alarming levels of PFAS (Per- and Polyfluoroalkyl Substances) in groundwater near industrial areas. These chemicals, once hailed for their utility, have now been linked to chronic illnesses, reduced immunity, and even hormonal disruptions. Rivers like the Yamuna, already grappling with untreated sewage and industrial discharge, now carry these invisible pollutants, amplifying the burden on ecosystems and communities that depend on them.

But forever chemicals don't stop at water. They seep into the soil, reducing its fertility and making crops less nutritious. They linger in the air, carried as tiny particles that settle far from their origin. And they quietly build up in our bodies, contributing to health issues that take years to fully emerge. These are not isolated incidents—they are woven into the systems that sustain our lives, and their persistence makes them one of the greatest regulatory challenges of our time.

India's regulatory framework struggles to keep pace with the scale of the problem. While policies exist to manage industrial emissions and agricultural chemicals, enforcement often falls short. Harmful pesticides banned in other countries are still in use, and untreated industrial waste continues to find its way into rivers and lakes. The gaps are visible in the widespread misuse of chemicals in agriculture, where farmers often lack access to safer alternatives or awareness of their long-term effects.

Take the example of pesticides. A farmer spraying his crops may not realize that the chemicals he is using could linger in the soil for decades, reducing its ability to support future harvests. This isn't a failure of intention but of support—outdated laws and limited access to education leave many unaware of the alternatives available. Meanwhile, unchecked industrial emissions contribute further, with factories discharging untreated waste into nearby water bodies, impacting not only the environment but also the livelihoods of those who depend on it.

Globally, countries are taking steps to address these challenges, implementing stricter laws and holding corporations accountable for their environmental impact. There's much to learn from these efforts, not to mimic but to adapt to our own context. India, with its vast agricultural landscape and growing industries, has the opportunity to lead with solutions that are rooted in its unique strengths—empowering communities, promoting innovation, and aligning with the cycles of nature that have sustained us for centuries.

The challenge is immense, but the path forward begins with awareness and action. Recognizing the unseen threats in our water, soil, and air is the first step toward creating systems that protect what matters most.

The Need for Policy Reform

The challenge may seem overwhelming, but the solutions are within reach. While individual actions make an impact, lasting change requires strong, thoughtful policies that guide industries and communities toward better practices. Policies have the power to reshape systems, incentivize innovation, and ensure accountability where it matters most. When carefully designed, they don't restrict—they inspire progress.

Take the example of harmful chemicals that persist in our environment. Around the world, countries have taken decisive action to phase out substances that pose significant risks to health and ecosystems. The European Union's restrictions on glyphosate, a widely used pesticide linked to soil degradation and potential health concerns, stand as a strong example. Similarly, the United States has made strides in reducing the use of PFAS in products like firefighting foams, recognizing their long-term impact on water sources and human health. These measures show what's possible when policy aligns with science and public welfare.

For India, the path forward lies not in imitation but in adaptation. The agricultural sector, the backbone of so many livelihoods, offers immense potential for transformation. Harmful pesticides and chemical fertilizers, while providing short-term gains, leave behind a legacy of depleted soil and polluted water. Banning the most damaging substances is a necessary step, but it must be paired with robust support for alternatives. Subsidies for organic farming, for instance, could make sustainable practices accessible to farmers, allowing them to care for their land while maintaining productivity. Imagine an agricultural landscape where the soil grows richer with each season, crops thrive without toxins, and water sources remain clean for generations to come.

Industries, too, must be held accountable for the waste they generate. Better monitoring systems to track industrial emissions and chemical disposal are essential. These systems need to be backed by strict penalties for violations and incentives for companies that innovate responsibly. For instance, packaging industries could be encouraged to shift toward biodegradable materials, with subsidies for businesses that adopt plant-based alternatives. Natural pesticides, derived from neem or other indigenous resources, could become standard practice, replacing synthetic chemicals that harm more than they help.

This shift is not theoretical—it has already begun in places like Sikkim, where state-driven policies have turned the region into a model for organic farming. By promoting chemical-free agriculture, the government has not only improved environmental health but also enhanced the quality of life for farmers and communities. This success story proves that policy can be a powerful catalyst for change, especially when it aligns with the needs and strengths of local populations.

Stricter regulations don't have to be seen as barriers; they can act as guiding principles that encourage industries to innovate. Companies around the world are already rising to the challenge, creating solutions that balance functionality with sustainability. From biodegradable plastics made of plant fibers to natural pesticides that work in harmony with ecosystems, these innovations demonstrate what's possible when creativity is fueled by responsibility.

Encouraging collaboration between policymakers, industries, and communities allows us to create a framework where progress doesn't come at the planet's expense. This is not a choice between economic growth and environmental protection—it's simply finding a path where both thrive together. This balance requires commitment at every level, from the fields to the factories, from the kitchens to the boardrooms.

The need for reform is clear, but so is the potential for a future shaped by thoughtful, effective policies. These changes will not only address the immediate threats posed by harmful chemicals but also pave the way for a healthier, more sustainable world—a world where harmony with the environment is no longer a choice but a way of life.

The Role of Government and NGOs

Collaboration between governments and communities has always been the cornerstone of meaningful change. While policies can set the direction, it's the collective effort of individuals, organizations, and industries that ensures progress reaches every corner of society. A government initiative gains strength when it partners with those on the ground—NGOs, activists, and local leaders who understand the pulse of their communities and can turn lofty ideas into actionable realities. Together, these collaborations create models of change that are not only impactful but deeply rooted in the lives they aim to improve.

Think about the story of waste management in urban slums. In a neighborhood once overwhelmed by overflowing bins and clogged drains, an NGO worked alongside local municipal bodies to introduce a waste segregation system. They started small—distributing color-coded bins for wet and dry waste, training residents on how to compost vegetable scraps, and ensuring that recyclables found their way to collection centers.

The government provided infrastructure and logistical support, while the NGO focused on education and building trust. Within months, what had once been a chaotic, unhealthy environment transformed into a cleaner, healthier space. The effects were visible—not only in the improved hygiene but also in the sense of pride and ownership residents felt toward their neighborhood.

Partnerships like these extend beyond waste management. Public-private collaborations have been instrumental in promoting sustainable agriculture and clean energy. In farming communities grappling with soil degradation and dwindling yields, joint efforts have introduced practices like crop rotation, natural pest control, and solar-powered irrigation systems. These projects empower farmers with tools and knowledge while providing financial support to ease the transition. The results are often transformative: healthier crops, lower costs, and fields that thrive year after year without exhausting the land.

One of the most inspiring examples comes from lake and river clean-up initiatives. Take the efforts to restore life to lakes and rivers struggling under the weight of pollution. NGOs leading these campaigns don't work in isolation—they partner with local governments to set up sewage treatment plants, enforce stricter regulations on industrial waste, and mobilize communities to stop dumping garbage into water bodies. These clean-up drives often start with volunteers removing visible trash, but their true success lies in raising awareness. Schools, religious groups, and businesses come together, united by the shared goal of protecting a resource that sustains them all.

Education plays a key role in making these collaborations effective. People cannot act on what they don't know, and raising awareness across diverse populations requires approaches tailored to their realities. For a farmer, this might mean a hands-on workshop demonstrating how compost improves soil fertility. For urban residents, it could be a sustainability drive showing simple ways to reduce waste at home or replace single-use plastics with durable alternatives.

The message doesn't need to be complicated—it needs to feel relevant and actionable.

NGOs have been champions in this space, bridging the gap between policy and practice. Many have created programs that take these ideas to the grassroots, whether it's teaching rural communities to harvest rainwater or equipping city dwellers with the skills to start balcony gardens. These initiatives not only address immediate challenges but also empower individuals to feel part of a larger solution.

A workshop on composting is a lesson in waste management, but it is also a reminder that everyone, regardless of their resources, can contribute to a cleaner, greener world.

Imagine the impact of this collective effort: government policies providing structure and resources, NGOs mobilizing and educating communities, and individuals taking small, meaningful steps within their homes and neighborhoods. Each piece of this puzzle strengthens the others, creating a cycle of support and progress that reaches far beyond what any one group could achieve alone.

Change doesn't always start with sweeping reforms—it often begins with a conversation, a shared goal, or a simple act of care. And when these efforts are nurtured and scaled, they build a future that feels both hopeful and within reach.

Creating a Framework for Natural Living

When these efforts begin to take root, they create a momentum that transforms more than the immediate problem—it shifts how we think, live, and care for the world around us. It's this collective momentum that can lay the foundation for a framework where natural living becomes the norm, not the exception.

Imagine policies that don't merely react to environmental damage but anticipate and prevent it. Policies that protect rivers before they turn toxic, support farmers before their soil is depleted, and guide industries toward sustainable innovation instead of waiting for harm to occur. These aren't distant ideals; they're steps we can take now, beginning with small but meaningful changes.

One place to start is mandating natural alternatives to harmful chemicals. Take the agricultural sector, for instance. Farmers often rely on chemical pesticides and fertilizers because they're affordable and accessible, but these come at a hidden cost—to the soil, to water sources, and to their own health. Policies that provide subsidies for natural alternatives, like bio-pesticides made from neem or compost-based fertilizers, can empower farmers to make choices that are both sustainable and effective. When supported by training programs that teach these methods, the shift becomes more achievable, creating healthier fields and richer harvests.

Beyond agriculture, industries like textiles and packaging hold immense potential for transformation. Funding research into biodegradable fabrics or plant-based packaging materials can help industries reduce their environmental impact while staying competitive. Imagine shopping for clothes made from bamboo fibers or receiving parcels wrapped in materials that decompose naturally—choices that feel good because they do good.

But even the most well-intentioned policies need enforcement. Stricter penalties for industries that violate pollution norms send a clear message: harming the environment is not an acceptable cost of doing business. This isn't about creating obstacles but about setting a standard that rewards responsibility and innovation. Industries that find ways to reduce emissions, recycle water, or minimize waste should be celebrated and supported, not treated as exceptions to the rule.

Now, think about what happens when these policies come together. Imagine rivers like the Ganga or Yamuna running clear, their waters supporting both marine life and the communities along their banks. Picture air carrying the scent of flowers and rain instead of smog and chemicals. Envision soil so rich and fertile that it nurtures crops season after season, feeding families with food that is fresh, nutritious, and free from harmful residues.

The impact extends beyond nature—it touches every aspect of life. Families would breathe cleaner air, drink safer water, and eat healthier meals. Communities would thrive, empowered by knowledge and opportunities to live in harmony with their surroundings. Industries would lead with innovation, proving that economic growth and environmental care are not opposites but partners.

This isn't a distant dream—it's a future waiting to be shaped. The rivers that run clear, the soil teeming with life, and the air carrying the scent of rain and renewal are not far-off ideals but possibilities shaped by the choices we make today. Every decision, no matter how small, becomes part of something greater, feeding a cycle of care that nurtures the earth and the people it sustains. It's a shared journey—a collective effort where governments, industries, and communities walk hand in hand.

Pause for a moment and look at the world around you. The soil under your feet, the water you drink, the food you prepare—all are quiet reminders of the earth's constant giving. But what happens next depends on how these gifts are honored. It's in the way a broken pot is repaired and repurposed instead of discarded, in the act of planting a single seed in a corner balcony, and in the care taken to choose what nurtures rather than harms.

Throughout these pages, we've explored the intricate connections that bind life together—the cycles of nature, the costs of convenience, and the beauty of living thoughtfully. These lessons are not abstract; they are woven into daily routines, into the very fabric of life. They are in the way food is grown, shared, and cherished. They are in the stories told by the things we mend and the choices we make. They are in the quiet moments when a leaf falls to the ground, ready to return to the soil that gave it life.

As you close this chapter, think about what you can do to carry these lessons forward. Start small, with the changes that feel natural. Swap a plastic bottle for a reusable one. Support local farmers at your nearest market. Learn about the policies and raise your voice for those that protect the environment. Join hands with neighbors to compost, recycle, or plant a garden. Each action you take is part of a larger story—a story of renewal, balance, and care.

And beyond the small steps, remember the power of advocacy. Support initiatives that align with the vision of a sustainable future. Encourage businesses and policymakers to prioritize innovation and accountability. Share what you've learned with others, creating conversations that inspire awareness and action.

Change doesn't happen overnight, but it begins with the willingness to act, to question, and to dream of something better.

This isn't the end; it's the start of something enduring and meaningful.

A chance to reconnect with the rhythms of the nature our - earth and to build a world where progress and preservation go hand in hand. It's a call to see yourself not as a bystander but as a changemaker, someone whose choices and efforts extend outward in ways you may never fully see but will always feel.

The earth has always given us its best—its soil, its water, its air. Now, it's our turn to give back. By embracing thoughtful practices, advocating for meaningful policies, and joining hands with those around us, we create a legacy worth leaving behind. A legacy where future generations inherit not only a planet that sustains them but one that thrives, enriched by the care of those who came before.

This is the story we can write together—a story of hope, resilience, and balance.

And it begins with you.

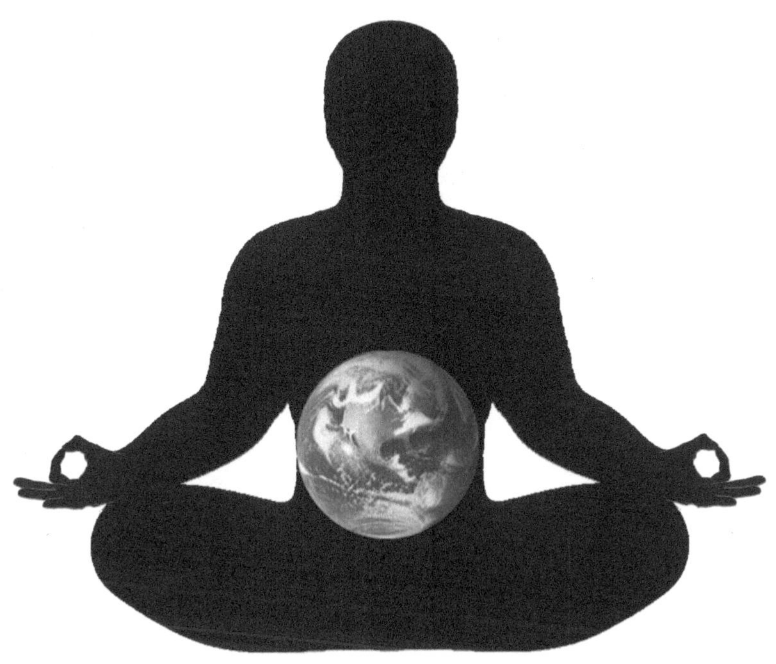

HARM *Less*

www.ingramcontent.com/pod-product-compliance
Lightning Source LLC
LaVergne TN
LVHW041211150826
845673LV00001B/364

* 9 7 9 8 8 9 6 3 2 8 1 1 7 *